TEN
WAYS
NOT TO
COMMIT
SUICIDE

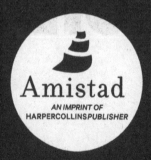

Amistad

AN IMPRINT OF
HARPERCOLLINS PUBLISHER

TEN WAYS NOT TO COMMIT SUICIDE

A MEMOIR

DARRYL "DMC" McDANIELS

WITH **DARRELL DAWSEY**

A hardcover edition of this book was published in 2016 by Amistad, an imprint of HarperCollins Publishers.

HarperCollins books may be purchased for educational, business, or sales promotional use. For information, please email the Special Markets Department at SPsales@harpercollins.com.

FIRST AMISTAD PAPERBACK EDITION PUBLISHED 2017.

Designed by Suet Yee Chong

Library of Congress Cataloging-in-Publication Data has been applied for.

ISBN 978-0-06-236878-2 (pbk.)

17 18 19 20 21 LSC 10 9 8 7 6 5 4 3 2 1

To my wife, Zuri, and my son, D'Son—the two main reasons for me not to commit suicide

CONTENTS

CONTENTS

TEN WAYS NOT TO COMMIT SUICIDE

ONE

UNCHAINED MELAN-CHOLY

EALING WITH DARKNESS, DEPRESSION, AND A DEATH WISH

For years, I hated waking up.

You hear me? Fucking hated it. It wasn't about shaking off the remnants of sleep. It wasn't about facing up to the regrets of the night before or the creeping anxiety about the unknowns of a new day. My hatred dwelled always in being in the then, the there. I didn't want to be awake or near anyone. In fact, I just didn't want to be.

From about 1995 through the early 2000s, I wrestled with deep depression, thoughts of suicide, and a relapse into the alcohol abuse I thought I'd left behind years earlier. During that time, my being awake meant struggling to be me for one more day. It meant grappling with the pain and uncertainty that I felt had come to define my life. It meant another day of the sort of quiet, desperate frustration that had seeped into my soul at a time when most people figured

I should be basking in the glow of a life well lived. My depression came in the form of being disappointed by the life I had created for myself. I was surrounded by "friends" I felt did not care about me. My voice was giving out on me. I felt empty inside. And as bad as all this was, it didn't compare with the most traumatizing blow in my life—a revelation that rocked me to the very core of my identity: in 2000, I found out I was adopted.

I had been damaged—and been damaging myself—well before I got that news, however. Depression had been shadowing me for at least a half decade by then, forcing me to endure a stomach-churning turbulence of mixed emotions that seemed to explode and whirl and collide inside me almost from the moment I opened my eyes. One minute I was angry. Then regretful. Then resentful. Then scared. And depressed, always depressed.

My constant companion, depression had crept in from seemingly every direction over several years of my life, a dark and indelible ink spread like graffiti along the crumbling walls of my battered psyche. Waking up meant facing those walls yet again, watching the cracks in them spread, and knowing that there wasn't a damn thing that I could do about it. And worse, that there wasn't a damn thing I wanted to do about it. To me, waking up just meant that I wasn't dead yet. That's how it came to be that, for nearly five years of my life, I contemplated killing myself almost daily.

Most of us wake up, roll out the bed, and get on with

our day. But for others, it's an everyday struggle to face life. All over the world, hundreds of thousands of people grapple with thoughts of ending their life by their own hands. They've given up, surrendered to the pain of a tragedy or the darkness of depression, or the aches of a physical ailment. They see no way out other than through death. Back in the day, I was similarly blinded.

I suffered all this in silence, which is the worst thing to do if you want relief. I avoided people, because I wanted to make sure that nobody really knew what I was going through. I didn't know how to express my pain, my anger. Not only did I bottle up my feelings, but I also made sure that I kept myself far enough away from everyone, regardless of whether they loved me or not, so that nobody could ever get an accurate gauge on how deep my despair ran. I withdrew into isolation because I couldn't cope with the anger and frustration that were driving me to want to hurt myself. I'd convinced myself that, whether I articulated my hurt or not, the pain would never go away. Just as crazily, as with many people who are suicidal, I actually thought I'd be doing the people around me—and myself—a favor if I committed suicide.

The biggest reason for my withdrawal was my vocal troubles and the problems that stemmed from them. While I was afraid of what it'd mean to lose my voice—who needs a rapper who can't rap?—part of my depression was rooted in not knowing why my voice had deteriorated. It wasn't until 1999, after a battery of tests, that doctors even figured out that I suffered from a rare form of spasmodic dysphonia. Most people with the condition experience vocal cord spasms when their voice box either contracts or expands. For whatever reason, *my* throat spasms when my vocal cords do either.

Even before doctors diagnosed the condition, though, I knew enough about it to believe that it had made me useless. I couldn't rhyme. All I could do was stand around wearing a fuckin' hat. I was embarrassed, and being dragged around the world to promote remixes only worsened my self-esteem.

Isolation was the absolute wrong move. It was potentially deadly in those moments because it ensured that my voice—the one feeding me negativity and promoting the notion that I lacked self-worth—was the only voice I allowed myself to hear. In those moments, it was precisely the last voice I needed to listen to. In those moments, I needed to realize that I wasn't alone.

I didn't want help, because I didn't think it was possible. My vision was skewed. My sense of time was disrupted. The pain I had experienced over the course of my ordeals became the defining struggle of my entire life. Nothing I had done mattered. I didn't think the wounds would heal.

To the world at large, I'm DMC, right? Rap star. Legendary MC. The Devastating Mic Controller. The King of Rock. One-third of Run-DMC, one of the greatest rap groups ever. But I feared that that part of my life had come and gone—and with it, much of my sense of direction and purpose. Whenever I looked ahead of me, all I seemed to see was emptiness. There was nowhere else for me to go, nowhere else it seemed I wanted to go. I just wanted to go back to sleep. For good.

I HAD UPS and downs over many years, but I was probably at my suicidal worst back in 1997, during a two-week-long tour in Japan to promote Jason Nevins's version of our classic "It's Like That." By then, my voice was long gone; Run-DMC had become irrelevant to many young hip-hop fans; and it was clear to me that our group, while still together in name, was over for all intents and purposes. I wasn't even thirty-five years old yet, and my life felt like it had crashed into a dead end. As a result, unbeknownst to anyone, I started planning ways to kill myself on that trip.

I had come to resent the group for any number of reasons. For years, probably beginning after our third album, the others had rejected almost all of my creative input. Worse, I felt, and still suspect, that the problems with my vocal cords were the result of me having to shout over tracks to be heard clearly. Our producers intentionally kept my vocals lower than Run's in the studios.

We had fallen off. We hadn't recorded a great album

in more than a decade and, worse, had put out more than one really awful one. Jay, who remained my friend throughout, had decided to spend more time focusing on his own pet projects. Run was looking toward a solo career.

By 1997, we should've called it quits—or at least I should have. We should've gone out on some Beatles shit or broken up like Cream. But we didn't. And so there we were, a legendary group that had outlived its prime, its members no longer bonded together by creative commonality or a shared dream of stardom or even fundamental friendship. We were in Japan to promote our brand, make some money for showing up, do some press, and pretend to be anything other than a shell of what we once were.

I felt like I was being used. It seemed like, within the Run-DMC dynamic, they had a singular purpose for me, which was holding a spot. I did shows and interviews, and made promo appearances, but I didn't count for much else outside of that. In the two years since I had begun dealing with vocal problems, Run hadn't called me once to check on my health. No visits to the house. He didn't even pass word through any of our mutual friends or business acquaintances. Run-DMC was a cash cow and a security blanket to him, nothing more.

Jay and I were different. Our bond wasn't strained nearly as much—but it still had stress fractures of its own. Our conversations had grown shorter, and even though they were fraught with far less tension than my conversations with Run, my chats with Jay were still more about business than anything else. Yet still we had a special bond.

Why am I here? I kept asking myself during that promo tour in Japan. I was there to be paraded around for a couple of bucks. I felt like some kind of show horse. I didn't have a problem making money, but that trip sealed for me just how far we'd fallen as a group and just how useless I had (in my mind) become to everyone around me. I felt used, pimped, and dirty. Instead of just coming clean about the point of the tour, Jay and Run kept talking about making this trip "for the people." They kept pitching it as some feel-good trip meant to reacquaint us with our estranged fans and make us relevant to anyone who may have missed out on us back in the 1980s. I might've been too obsessed with my own problems to care, but Run and Jay never lost sight of business. They wanted that paycheck.

No matter how much they were paying us to be in Japan, I wouldn't have come had only Run called. In fact, he tried for weeks to reach me to discuss the trip, but I avoided him like a virus. Run called only when he wanted something, when he thought there may be some opportunity to wring a few more bucks out of the Run-DMC brand. It had been years since our conversations extended beyond what time I was showing up for rehearsal or whether I planned to wear the Godfather fedora that people still associated with our group.

I'd rather have been home, in bed, or at the gym than

in Japan. I wasn't even feeling music right then. I had been a music lover my entire life, grooving to a playlist that ranged from Harry Chapin to Gordon Lightfoot to Grandmaster Flash, and I had stopped listening to almost everything. The only song I listened to then wasn't a rap or rock song. It was a soft-pop ballad by Sarah McLachlan called "Angel." I'd first heard it after getting into a taxi in 1996, and the song had stayed with me ever since. Back then, it was the only song I listened to and the only song that I allowed to be played around me.

I cannot overemphasize how important that song was to me in the midst of my depression. "Angel" kept me serene even when every fiber of my person was screaming for me to lose it. As troublesome as life was, "Angel" made me believe that I could soldier through whatever I faced as long as I kept striving. Years later, I cut my own record with Sarah McLachlan—who, I found out later, was also adopted—precisely because the lyrics to "Angel" meant so much to me in my darkest hours.

> So tired of the straight line
> And everywhere you turn
> There's vultures and thieves at your back
> The storm keeps on twisting
> You keep on building the lies
> That you make up for all that you lack
> It don't make no difference

Escaping one last time
It's easier to believe in this sweet madness
Oh, this glorious sadness that brings me to my knees

For all the depression that weighed me down, "Angel" buoyed me. Whatever my hesitations about suicide, I sometimes think I would have done the deed easily if it weren't for that record.

I thought long and hard about killing myself every day in Japan. I tricked myself into thinking that my family might be better off without me. I considered jumping out of a window. I thought about going to a hardware store to buy poison to ingest. I thought about putting a gun to my temple and pulling the trigger. Whenever I'd listen to "Angel," though, I always managed to make my way back from the brink. That song literally helped save my life. The song made me feel that I wasn't alone. It gave me great comfort.

RUN ONLY INTENSIFIED my depression when, during a television interview not long after I started having vocal problems, he announced that Run-DMC was breaking up because "D. can't rap no more." Even though my vocal problems were publicly known by now, Run hadn't discussed a breakup with me or Jay. He just went out there to the media and said it abruptly. He should've just said that he wanted me out of the group. Instead, he made me feel like I only mattered to do the Run-DMC thing and without that, I was worthless to him.

We didn't break up right then, but I suspected Run was plotting to leave the group without telling us. Those suspicions were confirmed midway through '97, when my manager, Erik Blam, and I just happened to visit the offices of our label, Profile Records, one day to take care of some business. I bumped into an A&R executive, who eagerly mentioned that Run was working on a solo project. Profile knew I was having vocal problems, but nobody at the label had addressed it.

So when I saw this guy, he came up to me and Erik excitedly. He assumed that Run and I were close and that I already knew about the project. "You want to hear Run's album he's been working on the last three months?" My eyes went wide, but Erik played it cool. "D., don't say nothin'," he whispered. Then he turned and said, "Yeah, let's hear it." We went into an office, and the A&R guy put on Run's demo tape. There were like five, six records on the tape that Run had laid down. He'd done a record with Slick Rick and a few other people.

I didn't let the exec see, but I was stunned. Why did Run feel like he needed to do this without telling me? Bad enough that he hadn't let me put many of my rhymes on our own albums after the first couple of them. I had wanted to leave the group for a long time and I never had, because I didn't want to let Run and Jay down. This just gave me more of an impetus to go my own way.

I may not have been able to rhyme anymore, but I could still write my ass off. I wish Run could've said, "I'm doing this album. Go get your rhyme book." It could've been like what Dr. Dre did with the DOC, the brilliant West Coast MC who lost his voice in a tragic car accident but still wrote for Dre's label and artists.

Believe me, I got the message. I responded by retreating into myself even more. I intentionally started to separate myself from the group. I didn't eat at the same restaurants with them no more. I didn't stay at the same hotels. I was hurt that, for years, they'd been rejecting my lyrical ideas in favor of the shitty music we had been putting out.

I stopped caring. I didn't want to do anything, didn't want to go anywhere. I was an emotional wreck. Meanwhile, growing in popularity, rap was becoming more lucrative. Just when I couldn't rhyme, I would turn on the TV and see my peers using hip-hop to expand their business opportunities. At this point, everybody was doing liquor and clothing companies. I was hearing other rappers say, "When I'm forty years old, I ain't even going to be rapping anymore." I was happy for them. It brought me down only when I thought about my situation and began to make comparisons. It depressed me more. More than a few times,

I caught myself looking in a mirror, thinking, *Oh shit, I'm in my midthirties. Forty is right around the corner for me. What am I going to do?*

As I became more of a recluse, I didn't want no tours. No spot dates. No interviews. No guest appearances. I just wanted to be left the fuck alone. People in and around the group had to beg me to do stuff. "D., just come on out for this. They're paying us good money." They'd tell me things like, "Get the money and *then* be depressed" or "Do it for the people because they want to see you." The money and fame hadn't ever been what drove me. I loved *hip-hop*, loved being able to rhyme and rip stages. I had worked hard, had helped build this amazing kingdom. Now I was feeling like I was about to lose the only job I'd really ever had and was really trained to do. It got so bad that all I wanted to do was sit at home.

There was constant pressure on me to make these public showings. They wanted me to come out and be DMC, but it didn't matter to them that DMC was only a shell of what he used to be. That's when it hit me: *They're not letting it go. Fuck my voice problems. They're going to milk this cow until there's powdered milk coming out the udders.* It was that revelation that drove me into the worst of my depression.

At the time, I didn't fully understand all the feelings I was grappling with. I knew I was hurt over losing my voice. I was angry and resentful that, in this Run-DMC situation, I was being pushed to do all these things when they knew and I knew that I couldn't rap anymore. What was the point of dragging me over to Germany or Japan if I couldn't be who I was, who people expected me to be?

In addition, I felt a void, this sense that even with all that was going wrong there was something else not right in my life that I hadn't been able to fully understand. There was an emptiness I was feeling that I chalked up to my depression over the voice problems, but it somehow seemed deeper. I was suffering from having stifled myself for so long. I constantly felt as if I were on the verge of either exploding or imploding.

I was tired of the gloom that was fogging my brain; tired of feeling passé and meaningless, tired of worrying day in and day out that all I had worked so hard for was over. I was questioning the whole point of my existence. *Am I really just here to be DMC, the King of Rock?* And if that's all there was, I told myself time and again, then that shit was over now. It was just time to move on, not only from MCing, but also from this plane of existence.

I was deeply wounded that nobody seemed to care that I wanted to grow as an artist without being told do this or that. Everybody was saying the same thing: "Fuck it, D., go get the check." Run, who was starting to get heavily involved in his church back then, would tell me stupid shit like, "Go sit with the bishop."

The bishop who oversaw Run's church was about money, too, so I knew what he was going to say. He may talk some shit about "doing it for the people" but really what he means, too, is, "Go get that money."

I remember telling Erik, "If Run and them really want to do it for the people, then fuck it. Give all the money away. I don't care if it's for a million dollars. Give it all to charity." But I knew that wasn't going to happen. It was about money, and I was way too wounded to worry about getting paid. Going out there like I was, useless, was painful to me. It hurt. It's easy to just go along with something, but if it hurts badly to do a thing, then you shouldn't do it. I often hurt myself to get along with others. I'm social, and social creatures crave acceptance, even if it's from someone they know who doesn't respect them. I was as bad for that as anyone.

Money hadn't stopped me from falling into depression. Money wasn't able to hold back the thoughts of suicide that had tantalized me for five, six years. Money don't mean shit if you ain't right. It got to the point where Run or Russell would call and I wouldn't even answer. I didn't want them to even say my name.

Artistically, I was flailing. I didn't know what I was going to do next, but I couldn't keep doing what I was doing, because it was tearing me up. I'd reached the point where even when I agreed to go places and do a few show dates, during the off time I had to be as far away from the guys as possible if I was going to function at all. I felt alone and isolated, and I wanted it that way—then I wouldn't have to try to please anybody.

I knew Jay cared, and I knew other people around me—my best friend, Doug "Butter" Hayes, longtime homeboys like my man Runny Ray, my manager Erik—they cared, too. But I couldn't completely articulate what I was feeling. I wanted to go through this thing alone. I was trapped between people who just wanted to use me and milk me dry, and friends and family who, although they loved me deeply, couldn't fathom what I was facing.

Predictably, everyone around me tried to talk that money shit. "Let's get this check." We were already getting paid well, but so what? After each show, every tour, I'd wake up still hurting. We were getting six-figure paydays again. When we fell off with *Back from Hell* in 1990, we probably were getting $12,500, maybe $15,000 a show. Now our lowest payday was 50 or 75 grand. Still, every night I went back to my room and asked the same existential question: "Am I here just to be DMC?" Nobody could understand that money couldn't fix my larynx. Money didn't make the group or our label respect my desire or my ability to write, to contribute as more than just a silent partner in Run-DMC.

Near the end of our run, my resentment began to turn into reluctance. I remember back in 2001, they were trying to get me to come to Los Angeles for a video shoot for the *Crown Royal* single "Rock Show." I wasn't even answering the group's calls. Erik was out there already, so Jay pulled Erik to the side and asked if he could get me on the phone.

Knowing how I felt about Jay, Erik agreed to try. I remember sitting with my wife and looking at the phone, my wife telling me, "It's them." I replied, "Let it ring." This was about me asserting myself and finally owning my disdain for how I'd been treated.

When I didn't pick up, I think Erik called and left me a message. When I called him back, he explained that Jay wanted to talk. I was disappointed in Jay over how some things had unfolded musically, but he was still my man. If it had been anybody else, I would have hung up on Erik's ass. But it was Jay. I had to hear him out. As we spoke, Jay realized very quickly that trying to lure me with talk about how much money we stood to make wasn't going to go anywhere. I'm just like, "No, no, no, no . . . I'm not coming." So he made a more personal plea.

"Would you just do it for me?" he asked. "Don't do it for the label, don't do it for the money. Just do it for me." That got to me. Jay was my man, despite all we were going through. I agreed to show up.

It wasn't long, though, before everyone on set realized that the DMC who showed up in LA was a different DMC from the one they'd been used to over the years. I wasn't going to lie and posture for Run-DMC anymore. I was still a mess inside, but I was growing tired of pretending I was what I had been. Even though I was participating in the video, I wasn't about to act as if I was actually part of the song. When I arrived on set, I told the video director, "Here's what you're going to do for the video. I'm standing in the B-boy stance. You're going to go to Run rhyming; when it comes to the close, you're going to show me a little bit and go back to Run and then to me." They were going to have to live with that.

The video director really thought I was going to act like I was in the record. He said, "Can you run around and do . . ."

I cut him off abruptly, "I'm not rhyming on the fuckin' record!"

He was shook, like, "Oh shit."

We were done making original material after that. We would continue to tour to get the money, but the forces that had been threatening to pull the group apart for so long won out.

The next two years brought still more heartache— death, family turmoil, recording setbacks—that saw many of my worst feelings intensify. The turning point came in Las Vegas in 2004. After attending a show, I went back to my room at Caesars Palace and downed an entire fifth of cognac in a matter of hours, all by myself. Staring at that empty bottle, I realized just how silly I had become in my desperation. Here I was with a life that few could even dream of, rich and famous, blessed with a loving family and great friends, and I had allowed my inability to get a handle on my feelings to threaten it all. I wasn't just tired anymore; depression had exhausted me. I wanted to get off the emotional tilt-a-whirl and to find my way out of the shell where I'd spent the past few years.

In 2004, I enrolled in alcohol rehab, an experience that taught me to deal with not just my drinking, but also with the repression and the overeagerness to please that had defined my life. With the emotional work I did in rehab and the constant love and support I was getting at home, I began to recover. After years of wallowing in self-pity and frustration over my ailments, I now knew that a new phase of my life was coming. I was looking ahead to considerations of what I could do next.

I told the group up front that I wasn't interested in recording another single note of the music we were doing. I had grown tired of participating in a process in which I constantly felt overlooked and devalued. I wasn't in hiding anymore, and I wasn't going to bite my tongue any longer. My vocal cords may have been traumatized, but rehab had given me the tools to finally find my inner voice. After a while, the group understood that Run's shit-talking was for naught in trying to convince me to do anything. I was a different person and they had to approach me differently.

I had had enough of making records as a member of Run-DMC anyway. I was getting off that treadmill and no one was going to stop me this time. Run was doing his own thing. Jay was doing his own thing. I was still unsure of myself, my direction, whether I could build a life after Run-DMC. I wanted to try, though. I realized that I wasn't ready to die—but for me to live right, I'd have to counteract the misguided thinking that had driven me to my lowest point. It meant embracing and building on some of the hard truths about how I'd fallen so far.

TWO

YOU DRINK, YOU DIE

ESCAPING THE GRIP OF ALCOHOL ABUSE

TWO

I'm an addict.

For most of my early life, I smoked and snorted and guzzled my way through almost every day. I started smoking weed at about twelve and drinking at about thirteen or fourteen. It came to me naturally and I didn't even think much of it when I first began, as it started pretty innocently.

The first time I ever smoked was with my friend Nathan and my man Dexter. Dexter lived on the corner. He was about three years older than me. He was also super, super, super cool, and had a basement full of the best toys and sports equipment. Dexter was the guy who had the best bike, the best basketball hoop, and the freshest clothes.

On this particular day, he had a marijuana joint.

Nathan and I were looking at it like, *What the heck?*

Even though we knew what weed was—my older brother Alfred smoked—we'd never been close enough to it to have it offered to us before. We were curious as hell. Dexter lit it up and gave it to me and Nathan. We each took pulls off it and were instantly like, *Whoa*. It felt good. Real good.

I didn't experience any of the epiphanies that I had heard about others having. I felt calm, relaxed, and more aware of my surroundings than I normally was. Being high was all right.

Before that day, Nathan and I used to go to Dexter's house to play basketball and wrestle. He also had the AFX cars and tracks, the model train set with the houses and the trees. He had a little city in his basement. After the first joint, we still did those things, but we also slid next to Dexter and said silly shit like, "Can we get some more of that reefers?" He'd look at us like, "Stop saying it like that!" We didn't even know how to ask for it right.

Pretty soon, I found out the whole damn neighborhood was smoking the stuff. My friends even started to bring weed to school with them. We went to Saint Pascal Baylon Elementary School, which was a Catholic school. There we were at a Catholic school, getting high, showing up for class, and then getting high some more. In between classes, we ran downstairs to the basement to smoke, and then back upstairs and into class—reeking. The nuns had to have smelled it. I'm surprised I never got caught.

For all our little experimentation, though, we were

still normal kids. We weren't bad boys or thugs of any sort. We were just mischievous children in working-class Hollis, Queens, doing what a sizeable chunk of the rest of America was doing in the late 1970s—getting high.

Weed made me feel like someone other than who I was, someone other than the comic book–loving nerd with the straight-A report cards and the thick glasses I'd worn since second grade. The weed made me feel cool, like the older boys. We smoked it to be cooler or funnier. We wanted to step outside ourselves, to not be square-ass Darryl who went to Catholic school, or little Joey "Run" Simmons from Hollis.

Prior to smoking, I'd always felt a little awkward, like I stood out from most of my friends. I wasn't really that much different from them, of course, but to me it often felt like I was. We're all different in our own ways, as individuals, as families, as communities. But as a young man, I magnified my differences in my mind, making them stranger or worse than those that set my friends apart from me. I wanted to fit in as much out of the fear of being ostracized as from a burning desire to belong. Being left out meant being alone, being vulnerable. You see the strength in numbers and the stability in the ties that bind, and you want that wherever you can find it. If you've got it at home already, then you want it on the streets or at work.

What made me different was that I wasn't invited—or allowed by my parents—to hang out on the block with my friends. I entertained myself with racecars and trains or reading the next issue of *The Incredible Hulk*. My parents were stricter than a lot of the other guys' parents. I had to ask permission for everything and couldn't do a lot of stuff the other kids did. Smoking made me feel like I was part of the in-crowd. Until I started smoking, I never really had that feeling.

Weed smoking also was a form of rebellion for me. It was my way of saying, "All right, so, I have to be home when the sun comes down, can't leave the yard when I want, have to be in the house by eight thirty—but at least I can do this!"

My rebelliousness took another turn when I discovered that I liked beer even more than weed. My friends and I had started to drink a little bit. It wasn't much. We'd just grab a trey bag of weed and then ante up and get a quart of Olde English 800. I don't think they were even making 40-ounces yet. It was just quarts.

I loved beer instantly. Weed made me feel cooler, but alcohol gave me a confidence that I'd never experienced before. The weed, the quart of beer were our method of escape from the start.

By nature, I was attentive to my surroundings, listening to learn and looking to learn. The weed heightened my attentiveness. I started seeing stuff that, even though I was high, I realized could be dangerous or become a problem. I didn't know if it was my imagination, but weed made me say, "I gotta not get shot, not get our money taken. We got to watch out for the gang fight. I got to know if they start shooting which way to run." Everywhere I went I was casing the joint. Weed made me more paranoid as time went on. It also made me feel a little nervous and shaky. The alcohol took the edge off.

A quart of Olde English didn't make me feel like the weed did. The alcohol was way different. It made me adventurous and bold, and, at least to my mind, it brought out the best in me. It made me stronger, faster, better. It was like fucking liquid bionics or some shit. The alcohol made me feel like a monster.

It continued like that for years, even after I started getting into music. It was back in the early 1980s. Run had gotten this gig at Le Chalet in Queens, on Hillside Avenue. He asked me to do it with him. This was the very first time he'd ever asked me to do something like that. He was getting two hundred dollars to open for the rapper Sweet G—who would later make the hit song "Heartbeat"—so he promised me forty bucks if I'd perform with him at the party. He even worked it out so that I wouldn't have to worry about dealing with my parents after being at a party late into the night. He arranged for us to go on at like eight thirty, nine o'clock, which meant that I could be home by eleven. Cool.

I needed confidence to get on the stage. Run had it by the barrelful after his preteen years spent playing shows in clubs and parties around places like Bear Mountain, New York. I was scared as hell! I'd never DJ'ed or MC'ed in front of anybody except Run and my friends. Run or my boy Doug "Butter Love," they would bang on tables and walls with their fingers to make beats, and I would bust rhyme after rhyme—especially if I was drunk.

By the time I'd turned fifteen, I was such a heavy drinker that the only way anyone could actually get me to rhyme was to give me a bottle of beer. The alcohol was my truth serum. I became the life of the party when I got drunk. I would rhyme for hours, about anything. A couple of quarts of Olde English 800, and I poured out my soul through my lyrics.

That's what it took for me to rhyme in front of my friends, and my anxiety was tenfold when Run approached me about rhyming in front of total strangers. To get on-stage in front of people I didn't know? I was afraid that even the Olde E wasn't gonna cut it. I was thinking, *If I'm nice off of Olde E, what's going to happen when I do* this? I broke into my mother's liquor cabinet and guzzled half a fifth of Southern Comfort like it was Pepsi. After that, we went to Run's house and began drinking quarts of beer. We downed two or three bottles and then we headed to the party. By the time we arrived, I was pissy drunk.

And I was still terrified.

I'd never been onstage before. Where was I supposed to stand? How far should I hold my mic from my mouth so that I could be heard without sounding muffled? How was I supposed to interact with the crowd? What if I messed up my rhymes and got booed? What if I *didn't* mess up my rhymes and got booed? I was so scared that I pulled the drawstrings on the black hoodie I was wearing so tight that it created a small opening that made my face barely visible. I didn't want anyone to see me. Meanwhile, Run was looking at me like, *This motherfucker . . . You can't go onstage like that!*

Out onstage, I was leaning against the speaker, basically hiding, avoiding facing the crowd. I amped up on my rhymes. By the end of the night, I was thoroughly intoxicated and completely unaware of my surroundings. It was one of those blackout nights. When I woke up the next day, I didn't even know how I had made it home. When I saw Run again, he said I did great but told me, "Next time rap to the goddamn audience!"

Aside from my being drunk, my performance was good. It made me believe that I needed alcohol to give me the extra edge to get onstage and be a great MC. They were a nice combo, the alcohol and the music, a potent combination for a kid who didn't usually have a lot to say.

Over the next several years—through hit records and sold-out tours—drinking went from serving as my creative springboard to being my crutch. My drinking worsened with every successive album we recorded. When we started recording our first album, which came out in 1984, I was drinking a quart or two of Olde English a day. By the time we dropped our fifth album, *Back from Hell*, I was drinking entire cases of beer every day. There are twelve 40-ounce bottles in each case, which means I was drinking 480 ounces of malt liquor daily.

The confidence that beer initially gave me turned into a sad dependence. I didn't just want the beer as a way of having fun anymore. After years of guzzling Olde E, it became my security blanket, my narcotic, and my path to withdrawal from whatever circumstances, feelings, or people I wanted to avoid at the time.

Avoidance is the real danger from abusing drugs and drink. I was drinking to numb the pain that I found impossible to express in constructive ways. But my heavy drinking and doping didn't just anaesthetize me. It also distracted me from the deeper issues that compelled me to smoke and sip in the first place. I felt inadequate and relied on liquor to enhance some false sense of power or importance. My abuse definitely wasn't a help in giving me any real emotional tools to deal with my deeper feelings of worthlessness. All that drinking did was to make it that much harder for me to face my fears and to do the hard work of conquering them.

Men aren't supposed to be thought of as fragile, but the truth is, men break, too. Sometimes we fall apart easily, sometimes not so. Throughout our communities, we see street corners and homeless shelters and prisons filled with men in dire need of repair. We are drinking ourselves into early graves. We are wiping ourselves out in fits of rage and crack smoke. We are killing ourselves with needles and nicotine.

For too many of us, it's easier to self-medicate. We'd rather find fake comfort in looking away from our problems—or at least gazing at them through the fog of coke or cognac—than face up to the scars that life leaves on us. In urban communities in particular, we deal with a social environment that is more often belittling and reductive than empowering. We are constantly told that we aren't smart enough or capable enough, that we can't lead or build families or run businesses. We live in communities where even people who look like we do buy into myths about our inferiority.

I tried to tell myself that my drinking was some act of defiance, as if I was somehow spiting on the group by destroying myself. In truth, my substance abuse wasn't resistance, it was surrender. It was giving in to the hurt, the confusion, and the rage. Alcoholism didn't drive me to introspection, but rather made it easier for me to hide from myself and from the truth about how low I felt.

By 1990, I was a full-blown alcoholic. You never saw me without a 40-ounce either in hand or nearby. It had gotten so bad that I installed a custom-built freezer in my SUV to have cold Olde E handy. When I walked around, I had someone in my crew carry a portable freezer that held my 40s.

I was nearing my breaking point. Until then, my drinking may have contributed to some social and professional issues—bad studio sessions, erratic behavior, repressed feelings—but I'd always been able to ride out those types of problems. I'd get fucked up. Do some wild shit. And then be right back at it the next night. Some days, I would leave my house twelve thirty, one in the afternoon, and not come home again until like three, four, four thirty in the morning. I'd be drinking 40s all day, come home, take a quick shower, and then go to the club, drinking Bacardi and Coke and screwdrivers and Olde English. When I was ready to leave the club I was still drinking on my way home. In my house, I would lie down for a second, get up, and start it all over again. I was hanging hard.

By 1991, the drinking had begun to take a toll on my body. I had picked up weight. I was bloated. I was suffering from bad bouts of the runs. There were probably three different occasions after *Back from Hell* when we were out on tour or doing spot dates and I would wake up with the runs. I mean, just stuck in the bathroom for long stretches, taking shits while in ridiculous amounts of pain. My stomach had started to feel like it was steeped in acid. Every time, though, the pain would soon subside and I'd be able to get back to performing—and drinking.

My drinking had grown so bad that I was barely eating. I wanted to drink so much that I didn't *want* to take time out to eat. How crazy is that? I would just drink all day. You know how hardcore drinkers often advise you to eat something before you drink? I was totally the opposite, because I thought, *The food is going to take away from the drinking episode. I don't want nothing to suck up my alcohol.* I wanted it to take full effect as fast as possible.

On one particular day when I woke up, the pain wouldn't go away. I got out of bed, stomach hurting, and I was saying to myself right off, "I better go eat." I went to the diner, had steak and eggs, hash browns, because I'm thinking, *You're burning the lining of your stomach. Get some food.* But the pain only grew worse with the food. I didn't know it then, but eating was probably one of the worst things I could've done.

I came home not long after that and got a call from my mother, who I'd been telling about the pain while I was on the road. I had figured I could deal with the pain because it always went away. Now it had gotten so bad that it hurt just to breathe. My mother told me to go to the hospital. Fortunately, there was one about five minutes from my house on Long Island.

By the time I got to see the doctor, the pain was severe. When he came into the examining room, I was doubled over and damn near in tears, begging him not to touch me. He just looked at me and nodded. I think he knew right away what the problem was.

"Do you drink, Mr. McDaniels?" he asked.

I nodded. "Yeah."

"How many cans of beer?"

"What?"

"How many cans of beer do you drink a day?"

"I don't drink cans. I drink 40-ounces."

His widened eyes said clearly what he was think-ing: *Who the fuck drinks a 40-ounce bottle of beer?* To a lot of people outside the hood, it's unheard of. Around the way, though, it was common. When you think about it, it is a crazy notion. Forty ounces of *anything* is not thought of by most people as a single serving. But in cities all across this country, young black people just like me were killing them-selves with 40s every day in our neighborhoods.

"OK, Mr. McDaniels," the doctor eventually said. "How many '40s' do you drink a day?"

I was like, "A case."

His eyes widened again. Surely he hadn't heard me correctly.

"What?" he asked.

"A case," I repeated. "I drink a case of 40s every day."

He didn't say another word to me. He turned around, waved to the nurse, and was like, "Admit this one."

They ran tests, took X-rays and EKGs and all that. When they finished, the doctor walked back into my room and said, "You can't go home, Mr. McDaniels."

"Hunh? Why not?"

"You've got pancreatitis—*acute* pancreatitis. Let's just hope your pancreas and your liver aren't scarred."

The diagnosis left me as stunned as it did scared.

I had been drinking beer since before I was in high school, running around Hollis with my little crew guzzling quarts of Olde E like it was nothing. When I'd switched over to 40s exclusively, around the time of our album *Raising Hell*, I figured it just meant that much more of the same. Drinking made me sociable and extroverted. Constant intoxication had become my haven, the buffer between me and the drama and resentment that were isolating me from the group and threatening to overwhelm me as part of Run-DMC. As crazy as it seems now, I had never once thought that drinking might actually kill me.

I was laid up in the hospital for a month and a half. For most of that time, I couldn't take anything orally, not food, not medicine, nothing. My only nourishment came from the IV bags connected to the long clear tube that had been jabbed into my arm. After the first month of liquids intravenously, they moved me to Jell-O, then soup. Eventually, I graduated to broccoli, fish, foods that would stay in my stomach. By the end of a full month, my doctor came around with good news.

"Fortunately, Mr. McDaniels, your pancreas and your liver don't show any scarring," he told me. "You'll recover." But with that good news also came a warning that would serve as my mantra for nearly ten years.

"You've got to stop drinking," he said. "This isn't ne-
gotiable. It's really just this simple. You've got two choices:
Don't drink and you live. You drink, you die."

You drink, you die.

I played those words over and over in my head. By the
time I was discharged from the hospital, they had sunk in
deep. *You drink, you die.* After that, I went cold turkey. I
no longer woke up shaking or had to fight off any demons
whispering in my ears at night. I didn't even crave 40s anymore. If I even saw a beer, my mind immediately went to
the doctor's warning. *You drink, you die.*

I WENT ALMOST a decade without having another drink,
and for a long time, it was like looking at the world through
another set of eyes. The world seemed like a brighter place,
more active, louder. Although I'd always credited alcohol
with fueling my confidence to perform, I discovered that I
could be just as powerful onstage when I was sober.

I performed sober for the first time ever in 1992, in
Germany. We were playing a lot of US Army bases back
then. We were in Hamburg. Traveling there felt different
this time. The hotels looked different. I'd been going to
the Marriott in Hamburg since '84, but now that I was
sober, I felt like I was seeing it for the first time. There was
shit in the lobby that I'd never noticed before. Suddenly, it
was like, "Where'd that come from?" "Was this thing al-

ways here?" The rooms looked different. The whole job was different—getting picked up to go to the show, the sound check. It was probably the same to everybody else because they smoked weed. But for me, without even a hint of a buzz off the 40-ounce, it seemed like it was all new.

When we hit the stage, it got even crazier. I was actually scared to death the first time I went out there sober. The music started. I grabbed the microphone. And then it seemed like, all of a sudden . . . the show was over.

The performance went by faster than I ever remembered any show going. I realized that when I was drunk onstage, it prolonged the experience. Everything seemed to take longer. Now that I was sober, it all seemed quick and easy. It was almost too easy, to be honest. I think that's when I first began to feel hints of boredom. It felt too routine, making me wonder whether this was really all there was to it. I think that was because I had all this creativity bottled up inside me, and I was out here speeding through the shows doing the same things I'd always done. I actually remember saying to myself onstage, *This is bullshit!* I don't even mean bullshit like it wasn't good, but bullshit like, *Is this all we're going to be doing? This is all I'm going to do for the rest of my life, go out and scream "King of Rock" and get money and get praise for starting the Adidas trend? I should be doing a new rhyme with a new beat.*

It was the perfect time to change things up, to bring that new creativity to the fore—but I wasn't able to utilize what I had in me. All through the early nineties, going to Switzerland and doing the Montreux Jazz Festival, I felt bored because I was sober. I was awake.

It was a wonderful feeling to have given up drinking, but I still hadn't learned how to deal with the issues that lay at the root of my addiction. Even though I wasn't numbing myself anymore, I was still evading the anxieties that were gnawing at me. I still felt rejected and disrespected by Run and Jay, who by this point were doing just about anything to stop the commercial free fall that had begun with *Back from Hell*. I still didn't know how to muster the courage to speak forthrightly about my feelings, fearing that I might come off as a complainer, as soft. Back then, I don't even think I ever spoke the words "I feel." I was still suppressing my spirit, even if I was no longer using beer to do it.

I recognized that I wasn't healed just because certain symptoms of a problem had gone away. The lack of self-worth that haunted me was very much present. My reluctance to express my feelings, to speak my own piece, remained strong. The sadness that I had tried to drown under gallons of beer and liquor continued to swim through my soul.

When I hit what was probably the roughest stretch of my entire life—the late 1990s to the early 2000s—it wasn't surprising that I eventually unraveled again. During this stretch, my life experienced some significant troubles. In

1995, I lost my voice almost entirely and had no clue as to why. In 1999, my doctors finally figured out the problem: I suffer from a throat disorder that causes my vocal cords to spasm randomly. The condition, they told me, was permanent.

In 2000, I had the fateful conversation with my mom and dad in which they revealed that I was adopted. My biological mother, as it turned out, had given me away as an infant, and no one had ever told me until then. After more than a decade of a rap career built on screaming my name to the world—*"I'm DMC/In the place to be"*—I discovered that I wasn't who I thought I was.

My whole life seemed like it was nothing but a lie. I was a rapper who could barely talk, let alone rhyme. Worse, my image of myself as part of the upstanding, middle-class McDaniels clan had come completely undone in one awkward conversation with my parents about my origins.

Depression had me firmly in its grip. Depression is an emotion that is slow and sneaky. It starts gradually, almost undetectable, and before you know it, you can't get out of bed. It affects people differently. For instance, some people want to eat everything they can get their hands on, while others completely lose their appetite. Some people sleep all day, while others can't get to sleep during regular sleeping hours. Depression is an overwhelming sense of sadness in which nothing seems exciting—even something you once loved. It causes you to feel shame. It paints everything in life with an overpowering sense of doom. It made me feel stuck, like I was running in place.

By 1995, '96, I began to grapple with serious thoughts of suicide. We were out on the road, and while everyone else was visiting sights or in their rooms resting, I was in my suite contemplating the many ways I could kill myself.

It wasn't long after that that I started drinking again. My relapse began during a stop in Germany in early 2000, at an Italian restaurant where I was dining with friends. Everybody was having a good time, laughing, joking, clowning around. Even the owner, drawn to the large group of guys seated at our table, had come over to introduce himself and join in some of the fun. He was a really nice guy and eager to get in good with us. Suddenly, he broke out an expensive bottle of wine and, unprompted, just started pouring wine for the whole crew. He had no idea I wasn't supposed to be drinking. He was just in a celebratory mood like everybody else.

He put a glass in front of me and started pouring. I sat there watching him. It was strike one. I should've stopped him then. I should've told him that I couldn't drink. I should've repeated to him the same words that had echoed in my head since I had been laid up in that hospital bed with pancreatitis in 1991: *You drink, you die.* Instead, I stayed quiet as he filled the glass halfway to the rim.

My friends weren't much help. To them, it was just one glass of wine. No big deal. They'd seen me go through four, five, hell, entire cases of 40s during my worst drinking days. I'm sure if my boys had suspected that one glass would hurt me, they'd have shut it down on the spot. When the restaurant owner started pouring, they noticed my hesitance but egged me on: "Come on, D., let's make a toast!" I should've ignored them and forcefully told the restaurateur no, but I used my being recently told that I was adopted as an excuse. I convinced myself that I was embarking on a new beginning, that I had found my true self, and that that was indeed good fortune worth toasting. All the pain, all the anxiety, all the fear of reigniting the pancreatitis that had kicked my ass nine years ago, suddenly seemed to melt away. *It's a celebration*, I told myself. It was strike two.

I lifted the glass, stared for just a second at the thick burgundy liquid sloshing around inside, and, for the first time in nearly a decade, took a sip of alcohol. *Put it down now*, I told myself. But then, just as quickly, I was telling myself, *Whoa, that's good!* I drained the entire glass and was ordering more. "Refill!" Before long, I was drunk.

Strike three. I was out.

Later that same night, we moved on from the restaurant to a nightclub, where the celebration continued. I ordered three, maybe four vodkas mixed with orange juice. The whole time I was scarfing them I told myself that because I was mixing the hard liquor with OJ, the drink was actually healthy for me. Like the wine and vodka, the lies I told myself went down easy.

The drinking continued over the next year. I tried on occasion to stop, but the willpower that I had mustered in the early 1990s and that had carried me through much of the decade failed me. I stopped for a week, just to prove that I could. I did—but I found myself craving a drink every moment, counting the days, hours, and minutes until that week was up. When my weeklong stint of sobriety ended, I fell back into the bottle harder than ever.

Pretty soon, I was drinking alone all the time, sneaking off from my manager, Erik, one of the few people who actually did admonish me about my excessive drinking, to down wine and worse. It wasn't 40-ounce bottles of beer anymore. As had hip-hop and the hood, I'd graduated to stronger stuff than malt liquor. Hennessey was the drink of choice now. I was all in, smashing pints and fifths of cognac with alarming regularity. Jack Daniel's and Jim Beam were names I got to know well, too.

When my wife, Zuri, realized I was drinking again, she was terrified for me. Even though I'd stopped drinking before we'd met, she knew very well that I had no business going anywhere near alcohol. "Darryl, you're killing yourself," she warned me over and over. "It ain't like you're somebody else and I'm saying don't drink because drinking leads to smoking. You can't drink, because you had pancreatitis. What do you think you're doing? Think of your son."

I lied and said my drinking was a "celebration" of my discovery that I was adopted. My wife saw through that and immediately exposed the heart of the matter: "No, you're drinking because you can't handle the news that you're adopted. You need to get help."

I was too consumed with my own issues to take her advice. In a matter of a few years, the life I thought I had secured had become unmoored from its foundation. I needed something familiar that I could actually control. In my mind, that meant drinking.

It was 2004 when I decided to get real with myself. My drinking was out of control and I needed help. I also needed to deal with the issues at the root of my drinking problem. I knew that being high wasn't the same as being in control—far from it, in fact. And if I was going to get real control over my life, I needed to confront my personal demons. I checked into a rehabilitation clinic in Arizona.

THREE

CAREER DECISIONS

OWNING MY TRUTHS, FORGING MY PATH

I was a liar.

Most of my life, especially early on, was spent hiding in the spotlight. Even as one of the most visible and sought-after musicians of all time, I squandered years, decades even, ducking my feelings. I was lying to myself and living in a state of fear. The world has known my name since Run-DMC first blew up the spot in 1983 with songs such as "It's Like That," "Sucker MCs," and "Rock Box." To hip-hop fans the world over, I'm DMC, the Devastating Mic Controller, the self-styled King of Rock, one-third of the most influential and popular rap group of all time.

To those closest to me, I'm just Darryl McDaniels, a dad, a brother, a husband, a friend. Whether you are a longtime pal from my old Hollis, Queens, neighborhood or a blood relative or one of the millions of screaming fans who've watched me prowl stages the world over, you've seen the real me revealed only in glimpses, in small portions. You've seen me perform over the past thirty years, but chances are you've rarely, if ever, seen who I really was. Lots of people know of me. Far fewer know who I am.

It's largely because, until fairly recently, I had no idea who I was. For a long time, I tried hard not to ever know. I went out of my way, in fact, to stay out of arm's reach of my own true self. I spent a lifetime crouched behind the haze of weed smoke, my face obscured by the upturned 40-ounce bottles of beer seemingly glued to my lips, my feelings hidden behind a four-eyed ice grill that could look out onto the world from the safety of tour buses and album covers without ever allowing the world to look in.

I was a liar.

I was a man out of touch with himself, someone who was able to lose himself behind the safety of his hooded sweatshirts amid the thudding beats of studio tracks and the screams of arenas full of fans. Rather than confront my feelings—or even those who hurt my feelings—I spent years pretending that nothing fazed me, that nothing was ever wrong. I aimed to please, even those—or perhaps especially those—who cared little to nothing about my own welfare.

As a Catholic kid growing up in Queens, I tried to be a model son, at least in my parents' eyes. To my big brother,

Alfred, I was the tagalong younger sibling eager to emulate him and his friends even when, deep down, I knew that what he wanted wasn't what I wanted. Out on the streets in Hollis, I did what I could to fit in with the other kids in my neighborhood, to be liked, to be cooler than I felt I ever actually was. I gave in to other people's expectations of me, bent myself to their perceptions. Before rap made me famous and for many years afterward, I stuck dutifully to the role of good soldier, loyal pal, and compliant coworker. I did what was asked. I went along to get along. The unnecessary burden of living a life of trying to please others, which is essentially impossible, nearly killed me.

MY INTRODUCTION TO hip-hop—the very thing that would one day make me rich and famous—came as a result of me giving up something I loved for someone else's desires.

Growing up, I'd always been a comic book geek. I loved to draw superheroes almost as much as I liked to read about them. Comics were an escape, a way to make myself feel strong and invincible rather than like the quiet little four-eyed nerd I essentially was.

Hip-hop culture has always been strongly influenced by comic books—comic books and kung fu flicks. For poor black and Latino kids growing up in places like the South Bronx, Harlem, Los Angeles, and Detroit, comics and karate movies represented a power fantasy, a chance to flex muscle that, as a social group, we didn't have much of in America. In hip-hop, we took on aliases like superheroes and borrowed titles like "grandmaster" and "grand wizard" from kung fu protagonists. Remember that illustrated cover for "Renegades of Funk" that looked like a Marvel comic, the one that featured Afrika Bambaataa and them busting through that wall? There was that Newcleus cover for *Jam on Revenge*. The Sugarhill Gang and Grandmaster Caz had rhymes dissin' Superman. So comics, kung fu flicks, and hip-hop have been down with each other for a long time.

I had a much closer relationship to one than the others early in my life. I dug the kung fu flicks, but comics were my real thing. The Hulk, Captain America, Iron Man, Spider-Man, the Avengers, the Defenders, those were some of my favorites. I was a big Marvel Comics guy, not really into the DC stuff. But I did like Batman. Batman was cool, dark. Superman was too commercial and the story line too wishy-washy.

My brother, Alfred, was the one who had gotten me into comics. He started collecting first—we wound up buying hundreds of comics—and not long after he started collecting, he started drawing over the comics, using tracing paper. He'd trace over Spider-Man, the Hulk, Captain America, and then he'd color it in. It was only a matter of time before I started doing that, too. Even after Alfred stopped, I kept going. Eventually, I got real good, to the point where I could just draw freehand.

When hip-hop started to come over the bridge from the Bronx to Queens in the late '70s, I wasn't thinking much about it. Although it was easy for me to see the MCs and DJs who played our park jams as superpowered figures showing off their cool alter egos, I was still heavy into the Hulk and Spider-Man. Hip-hop was just that new thing, something we did for fun, not meant to be taken too seriously. I wasn't even allowed to hang at the parties, because I was too young. I had to leave just when the DJs would be setting up, because I had to be home by ten.

The year following the US bicentennial, the scene exploded in Queens with break-dancing, graffiti writing, MCing, and DJing. The kids around my way, especially the older dudes like my brother, wanted to be part of it.

Back then, it wasn't even about rapping. The MC thing wasn't fully revealed yet. The big thing was DJing. My brother wanted to get turntables because that's what the dudes his age were into. They were chasing girls, going to the park jams, and hanging out all night. In those days, you had DJ crews all over Queens. Everybody wanted to be the DJ at the block party or at the house party.

I wasn't necessarily interested in the scene. I wanted to be an illustrator because comics were my real love. Me and my friends played with skateboards and model cars. I might've even still been playing with army men a little bit. We were twelve, thirteen, but my brother and his friends were like sixteen, seventeen, eighteen. They were drinking Bacardi and smoking weed (the *right* way).

All of my brother's friends wanted to be DJs. They started buying turntables. I remember that a guy in the neighborhood named Anthony was the first one to get some. Then a guy we knew named Boobie got some. One day not long after that, my brother came to me and said, "Yo, we got to get some turntables. We got to get some money."

I was one of those kids who really liked being a kid. I got along with my brother well and would sometimes go out of my way to win his acceptance. And I think both of us tried to impress his buddies. The bottom line is that Alfred and I were your classic middle-class black teens. We didn't sell drugs. We weren't stick-up kids. We weren't going up in nobody's house to rob or out on nobody's corner to sell. So how were we supposed to get money for turntables?

We were at the house, in Alfred's room. Getting turntables was all he'd talked about for several weeks. Alfred wanted a sound system and he didn't care what else he had to sacrifice to get it. As soon as Alfred mentioned getting money for turntables, I looked at him, and, in my mind, there was an image playing out like a movie. I had a vision of him saying we needed money and then me thinking, *No, no, don't say, "We gotta do a comic book sale."*

Soon as that thought goes through my head, Alfred pipes up and says, "We gotta do a comic book sale."

I was crushed. I lived for the day each week when the brand-new Marvel titles would hit the shelves at the drugstore around the block. Whatever little allowance Byford and Bannah McDaniels, our parents, decided to throw my way always managed to find its way into the hands of some merchant in exchange for my little slice of four-color, glossy-covered heaven. When last I'd seen Spider-Man, he was fighting for his life against Doctor Octopus, and I needed to know how the fight ended.

Alfred was older, and he was my brother. I looked up to him, loved him as much as he loved me. If he really wanted the turntables, I'd have to start surrendering some of my favorite comics, because making him happy just seemed to be the right thing to do, even if it left me a little mad.

We put up fliers around the neighborhood, spread the word to our friends about the comic book sale. We raised a lot of money. It seemed like all the guys in Hollis came over to buy comics. Joseph Simmons, a.k.a "Run," from Saint Pascal's, came with his friend Harold. I was in 7–2. He was in 7–1. It was the first time he had come over my house.

Alfred sold the comic books, bought his turntables, and began building a little system. He took a receiver, an amp, and the two speakers that we already had in our house. Later, the system became my mother and father's pride and joy. They used to use it during Christmas and at parties. You know how, as a kid, you'd stand at the top of the stairs at night to try to figure out what the adults downstairs were doing? We used to do that whenever we heard speakers blasting Al Green and Aretha. We knew it was a party. Of course, that's also when my parents would tell me, "Get your butt back in your room." In the morning, I'd go downstairs and find empty Johnnie Walker bottles and ashtrays full of cigarette butts.

It became my parents' party system. When Alfred first told them what he wanted to do in putting the system together, Byford and Bannah were amused. "I take this mixer thing and we play two records at the same time," my brother said.

Every now and then, they'd yell at us to turn the music down when we were in the basement banging away on the wheels of steel like those garage-band kids would be wailing on their guitars. Otherwise, that's as far as our parents' complaint went. I think their thing was, *Well, at least we know where our kids are.*

Alfred got *his* turntables. Typical of most older siblings who don't want their annoying kid brothers disturbing their things, he wouldn't let me touch them. I'd surrendered some of my prized possessions so my brother could play DJ, and he wouldn't share the fruits of my sacrifice! He and his friends would go in the basement and practice for hours while I had to either stay upstairs or stand on the periphery of his sound system and watch. The only time I got to spin was if Alfred was gone. It was during those occasions when I (alone, and later with Run) would sneak downstairs and try to mimic Alfred and the older boys I'd seen spinning wax and learning the rudiments of scratching and cutting.

The music thing was cool, but it wasn't what I really wanted. It was fun, but I still missed those issues of *Iron Fist* and *Daredevil* that I'd had to peddle. I'd tried to make myself want the turntables because Alfred coveted them so badly. But that wasn't my truth. I was lying and pretending just to keep the peace. But, at the same time, I was becoming a little resentful, especially since he wouldn't allow me to touch them.

As it turned out, I eventually fell madly in love with hip-hop, first as a DJ and later as an MC. I never lost my love for comics, but by the time I was in junior high school, hip-hop had become my obsession. Run and I had become closer in the years since he and the other kids had plundered my comic collection. Over time, he and I cultivated our love for rap together. We snuck into the basement whenever we could to play on that sound system, even after it started to get a little worn. Hip-hop was becoming my new haven, another alternate reality that I could slip into and pretend to be somebody, anybody, other than the quiet kid who got straight As at Saint Pascal's. Like many of the kids my age who were falling in love with hip-hop, I had segued from DJing to rapping. Meanwhile, Run, who Russell had had DJing gigs at age twelve behind a then up-and-coming Harlem rapper (and future legend) named Kurtis Blow, had also begun writing rhymes. I wasn't that serious about it. For Joe, hip-hop was a pastime and a future dream. Russell, an aspiring party promoter and record producer who was attending NYU, had met Kurt as a student there. Russell had promised Run that he could cut a record once he finished high school, sort of as an incentive for him to stay serious about his education.

Over the next few years, throughout middle school and high school, Run constantly reminded Russell of that promise. Once Run found out that I could rhyme, too, it wasn't long before he enlisted me in his dream. Even though Russell absolutely hated my voice and couldn't have cared less about what I wanted—I was just his annoying kid brother's equally annoying friend, after all—Run eventually got him to agree to put me on, too.

True to his word, Russell booked Run studio time shortly after he graduated high school and, that summer, Run and I recorded our first songs ever: "It's Like That" and "Sucker MCs." For Run, it was the realization of a dream he'd had since he was a tween. For me, though, it was just something to do before I headed off to Saint John's University that fall to pursue my college degree. I didn't even tell my parents that I had gone to the studio to record the songs. I didn't think they'd approve if I asked, so I just made up a story about hanging out at Run's house. I liked playing rapper, sure. But I had been raised in a practical, hardworking family that emphasized learning a skill and putting it to use to build a decent life. Music didn't seem to have any place in that scenario. After we laid down the tracks, I went back to my normal life. I moved on, preparing for college.

When I got to college, I hated it. Going there was what I thought I was supposed to do. I didn't know why I was supposed to want it other than that other people, my parents and school counselors and teachers, wanted it for me. I knew college could yield things, and I knew that, as an academic whiz from K through 12, I was expected to go. As a kid, I'd always wanted to attend college to play football, but that dream had died once I got to Rice High, a Catholic school that was a basketball power but didn't field a football team. My football dream had died on the vine quietly, without me so much as saying a word to my parents or anyone else about what I'd wanted. I felt deep disappointment over not being able to play, but I'd kept my mouth shut to my mom and dad. I can see now that early on, I had begun to master the art of suppressing my feelings in the face of other people's expectations.

Prior to college, I had always loved school. First day of ninth grade, first day of tenth grade, I looked forward to it. College was different. When I got to campus on my first day of college, I saw beautiful buildings. The grass was cut. Students were doing their college thing, sitting around studying on their way to their classes and whatever. They looked happy, but I was miserable. The bus ride by myself was miserable. Looking for the first class was miserable. The plan was for me and my friend Doug Hayes, who we called Butter, to go there together. It ended up that we didn't have any classes together and barely saw each other on campus. I spent a lot of time by myself.

In elementary school or high school, you may not know anybody on the first day, but by the fourth day you know people because you're in the same classes and the curriculum is designed for interaction, socialization. College is different because while you don't know nobody on the first day, it doesn't seem to change. College is competitive, grounded in individualism. You go to one class after another class, and you don't know nobody in any of them. Then you come the next day and you still don't know nobody. It went on for weeks in that manner.

I tried to adjust. I told myself that I had to grow up and that this is what people did when they left high school. I tried to keep myself interested. I started to think about what I could change my major to that could possibly make the experience enjoyable. I didn't find pleasure in my business-administration courses and I didn't even know what courses I liked. I knew I could draw, so I thought that maybe I would try architecture or graphic design. I hated those classes, too. I was also scared of not getting my degree—then what would I do?

Right around that time, Run called. He told me that Russell was shopping the record that we had made. He'd call every day, filling me in on what Russell was doing, telling me how he was taking our record to major labels. Kurtis Blow had been the first MC—not rapper—to be signed to a major label. Before that, rappers had been on Sugar Hill, a little independent label. Russell had gotten Kurtis a deal with Mercury Records. He figured he could do for us what he'd done for Kurt.

I saw that Run was excited. He was enrolled in community college. He came from an educated family. Russell had gone to college, which is where he had met Kurt. Run's father worked in the school system. Run was also focused on music. He saw what was happening with hip-hop. Kurt was killing. Kurt was touring the world, going to London. Russell was Kurt's manager, so his management was booming. Meanwhile, Run was doing more appearances with him. Run was getting gigs, coming home with tapes of the shows, bringing me Kurt's albums.

I wasn't into it. I was on a whole other plane of existence. My brother had enlisted in the army. Doug and I weren't hanging, because of our different college schedules. I was alone. I got by with my tapes, 40s, and weed. They were my relief from the world.

Second semester came around, and Russell finally landed a deal. Run called me, frantic. "Russell got us signed!" Russell had found some little label called Profile Records to take us on.

I still wasn't excited. It was cool and all, but that shit didn't mean anything to me. I was somewhere else. I was trying to figure out life. It's not that I was knocking Joe for being excited. He had worked hard for this. But my time in college had made me lonely and sad. I was miserable and wasn't sure that anything could make me happy. I wasn't even going to all my classes. I was cutting out and taking the bus from the campus to Hollis. I was simply displeased by not having a direction for my life. I didn't see music as an option. At the time, everybody thought hip-hop was a fad, so I didn't see it as a career.

Since Joe was my man and this was something he really wanted, I went with the flow. He got me to come to the city a few days after his call so we could start signing papers. First we had to sign with Russell, I guess because he had set up everything. Once Russell had those papers, Profile could close the deal with Russell.

A couple of days later, I was back home in Queens and I decided to talk to my parents about where my life was going. I was wasting their money at Saint John's, and I realized that I had to tell them something. I said, "Ma, I want to be happy. I like drawing so even if I wind up drawing the funnies, the comics in the local newspaper, that's what I'm going to be doing." My mother had always been upset at the idea of me drawing the funnies. My dad was cool with it. I just wanted to keep it real with them about my desire to live out my own aspirations—whatever they were.

I felt like a weight had been lifted off me. My parents weren't upset. They just wanted me to do whatever made me happy as long as I could make a living at it. Whatever I decided would be OK with them. There was a lesson in there that I wish I'd learned right then: I had shared my true feelings with them and it was fine. Nobody died. Nobody freaked out. It was my life, and they wanted and expected me to live it in a way that made me happy. If I had realized back then that speaking my truth didn't involve disappointment and anger from others, I may have made more genuine decisions later in life. I may not have spent so many years later shutting up and denying myself.

THE RECORD CAME out before I got the chance to have another conversation with my parents about school. I was home one day when Run called. "98.7 KISS-FM, they're going to play the record today at five thirty. Make sure you're listening," he announced.

I went back in my room. I got the radio out. I was doing some homework for one of those classes that I hated. I remember sitting there, not wanting to do it, but thinking, *Let me just get this out of the way.*

"It's Like That" came on the radio. It sounded just like it sounded: dense, empty, yet thick. It sounded so different from everything else that was out. I heard Run's voice first—"Unemployment at a record high . . ." I followed him. I thought how funny it was to hear my voice on the radio. It was ill. It was weird.

As soon as it went off, the phone rang. "You heard it?" Run asked excitedly. I'm like, "Yeah, I heard it. Cool." Run was screaming at the top of his lungs over the realization of a lifelong dream, and I sounded as if my dog had just been run over by a Volkswagen.

"It's Like That" debuted on a weekday. The weekends in New York were when the hip-hop DJs—Red Alert, Chuck Chillout, Mr. Magic—would play the new stuff. This was when we got to see whether our music was good for real. They played "Sucker MCs" on Friday. Then they played it again, like two or three more times. On Saturday night, they played it two or three times. Suddenly, they were playing both my songs on the radio.

As dope as I thought it was, as excited as I was when the song got airplay, my excitement remained tempered by my anxiety. I was sitting in the Rathskeller at Saint John's. It was where the students went to hang after class, to eat lunch and socialize. I was in there because I was cutting a class. Someone had a radio playing through the speaker system in the building, and "Sucker MCs" came on.

Dudes, girls—everybody in the lounge jumped up.

"Yo! This is the best song out right now." "Who are these dudes?" "Who is Run-DMC?" I was sitting there watching and thinking, *It ain't gonna last.*

I went back to moping.

A couple of days later, Run called again: "Yo, the records are a hit across the nation. Russell booked us a show. Pack your bags, D. We're going to do a show. North Carolina."

My mother and father were in the kitchen. "Hey Mom, hey Dad. Remember that time I came home at two thirty in the morning? Remember that night I came home late in the summertime? In August, and I said I was at Run's house? Well, I wasn't really at his house. We actually went to the studio and made a record. Now they're playing the record on the radio, and Run wants me to go to North Carolina for a show."

They just looked at me. The only records they thought mattered came from Motown.

"Oh, hell no. You get back up there and finish school." That was my mother. My father was just "No!"

I didn't say another word. I turned around and immediately went to bed. I thought that college was what I needed to be doing, too, no matter how much I didn't like it. But I didn't want to disappoint Run. He had worked hard, and not just for himself but for me, too. He had badgered Russell and had stayed on me about rhyming. I felt like I owed it to him to try my parents again. I waited a day and went back to them. I broke it down as honestly as I could.

"Mom, here's the deal," I said. "Let me go do this show and whatever money we get paid to do this show, I'll put it toward my school." I talked and talked and talked. After a while, they agreed to let me do the show.

"Whatever happens, don't just drop out of Saint John's. Call and take a leave of absence—but don't drop out," my mom said.

FOUR

CLOSED
CIRCLES

LIFE IS BETTER WITH SUPPORTIVE FRIENDS

FOUR

Run-DMC got hot fast. Our first album became the first rap album to sell more than a half million copies and earn gold certification from the Recording Industry Association of America. "It's Like That" and "Sucker MCs" became instant hip-hop classics. "Rock Box," the first rap single to marry hip-hop with rock, catapulted us to international fame. The video became the first rap video to get airplay on MTV. Me, along with Run and our DJ-producer, Jason "Jam Master Jay" Mizell, became certified stars out of the gate.

Rather than liberate me, our success only put more pressure on my shoulders. Run-DMC took on the feel of a high-stakes job. We were expected to continue the momentum we'd created with those first singles, even though we'd already done more than most of the groups that had come before us. We weren't just rapping for fun now. Run-DMC's success had been a boon for the label, for our friends who had started working for us as roadies and security, for Russell and the small management company he was building around us, and for Kurtis Blow. For my part, hip-hop was still a game, something I did as an escape, as a way of unleashing my otherwise-repressed personality.

Almost as soon as we began to earn major attention, the dynamics in the group changed. Run began to spend less time with the group and more time away with his girlfriend. Me and Jay hung together a lot. Over time, Run grew more and more emotionally distant. He was about business. Run had always been the front man of our group, and now that we were a hit, he was taking that job much more seriously.

When we were together, Run barked at me a little more, always nagging me about my wardrobe ("D., you bring ya hat?") or our routine ("Don't ad lib out there. Just do it like we rehearsed"). But Run had always been a bit of an anxious type, always fearful that something was going to go wrong. He wasn't a tyrant, just anal as hell. It annoyed me, but I was still having enough of a good time that I was willing to charge it to the game. He'd scream at me, or bark some order at me, and I'd blow it off and look the other way. I wasn't confrontational. Plus, Run was my friend, and he meant well, right? *It doesn't bother me*, I'd tell myself. *Whatever.*

Many men are like me in this regard. We've always got to pretend to be invulnerable, to be above any sort of emotional pain, particularly in areas of friendship. I was expected to be stoic and undaunted in the face of whatever pressures came my way. In truth, it bugged me. I was lying like hell to myself about it the whole way, refusing to admit that Run's barbs and the inexplicable distance between us stung. I felt wounded, sad, and disappointed. I believed that my bandmates didn't take me seriously. Rather than address my feelings of inadequacy, I drank, smoked weed, and found other ways to anesthetize my spirit.

The group afforded me the opportunity to express my creativity. I was a prolific writer with reams and reams of material. As long as I felt I was able to bring my music and my ideas to the table, I was willing to put up with Run's behavior.

Our first album had won over fans from coast to coast and overseas. Our success had put me in proximity to many of the same rappers I'd idolized for years. At home, though, the reception we were getting from some of the other rappers was anything but warm. When we blew up, a lot of the rappers that came before us started hating. In my mind, I had been taking these dudes out for years, slaying them in epic rap battles that had played out in the solitude of my mother's basement in Hollis.

In many cases, the resentment came from rappers who I'd always looked up to, but I didn't take any of it personally.

MCs are innately competitive, showmen who maintain a take-no-prisoners attitude when it comes to rocking a party or a concert. The MCs who had come before us weren't about to just lay down and surrender their spotlight—not the MCs who had come out of the club scenes in Harlem, and certainly not the rhymers who hailed from the Bronx, where rap had been born.

Their grudges had absolutely no bearing on how I felt about them. One thing about me was that I may not have been honest about the negative feelings I'd harbored, but I have never had any problem expressing my genuine feelings about things I love.

I think showing love is an important part of being true to yourself. Too often, we worry about the response of others. I was constantly fretting over what people would think about critical remarks, but I wasn't much concerned with showing praise. In those instances, I've never been able to contain myself. Getting past the need to conform to others' desires allowed me to live from the inside out and not the outside in, to start with myself and what I think and feel. In those moments I didn't sacrifice my own desires for fear of someone's reaction.

Being DMC put me in the same room as guys like Grandmaster Caz and Melle Mel and the Treacherous Three, all MCs I had come up listening to even before Run and I had ever cut a record. It was a pleasure that I embraced every chance I got. I acknowledged others without shame or reservation. I wasn't too cool or too standoffish.

On "Jam Master Jay," for example, I wrote: *"We're live as can be, not singin' the blues / We came to tell y'all all the good news / The good news is that there is a crew / Not five, not four, not three, just two."* It was inspired by the Cold Crush Brothers. It was also me going at my other favorite groups—the Furious Five, the Funky Four Plus One More, and the Treacherous Three. I'm throwing in lines like, *"It's about time for a brand-new group / Run-DMC to put you up on the scoop."* When competing groups heard it, they instantly understood. As I got to know the other groups, I actually felt bad at times for having called them out like that.

Run-DMC was out on the road a great deal. In response to my lyrics, I saw some of hip-hop's most legendary MCs diss Run-DMC right to our faces when I went to clubs. The first Fresh Fest tour had us on the same bill as the other hot new groups, but it also featured Kurtis Blow, who, even in 1984, was considered the king of rap. Kurt had problems with us. He resented our success, same as the others. We were busting his ass onstage every night!

Aside from us rocking it, many people were hating on us because we weren't housing-project hard rocks who had come up grooving at park jams with DJ Kool Herc or Afrika Bambaataa. People were like, "Who the fuck are these suburban, middle-class kids from Queens?"

After we got home from the Fresh Fest tour, I started

to hear a little more of the grumbling. A few songs came out that took shots at us.

Once we did an appearance at Columbia University. It was just me and Jay that day because Run was sick. Jay actually had a broken ankle, from playing basketball, but he went up there with me anyway. After we arrived, we went to the dressing room and waited to get word about the show. While we were waiting, who comes walking in? The badass Cold Crush!

The only thing going through my mind was, *Oh shit! Oh shit! There go Caz and JDL!* I had never seen them in person before, and as far as MCs went, they were the gold standard. Cold Crush had been my inspiration, the group that had made me step away from the turntables once and for all and pick up a microphone and a pen. As a student at Rice and Saint John's, I had lived for—and through—their music, especially their cassettes. I wanted to tell Caz how I'd taken the nickname DMC after he'd made three-letter names popular. I wanted to tell them how the fire they had been spitting from as far back as the 1970s had so thoroughly ruined me for the pop rappers who had come after them. This was the Cold Crush, and I thought that these guys were the greatest group ever. I didn't give a fuck if I was in Run-DMC. I was a fan!

They walked into the room, then, as soon as they saw it was us, they swerved! I mean, they turned right around and walked straight back toward the front of the dressing room. The MCs never said a single word. Me and Jay were sitting while all four of them were standing near the door with their arms folded and their backs to us. We were straight getting dissed!

Eventually Jay started talking to Charlie Chase and Tony Tone. DJs are like our old producer Larry Smith and those other musicians; they always know each other, always talk. Even if two rap crews are beefing, it's like the DJs are the diplomats, the ones who are allowed to still deal with each other. But the MCs? Oh, hell no. Caz and JDL ain't have shit to say to my ass that night.

I ain't give a fuck! Yo, I just got dissed by Cold Crush! That shit is dope!

There were other incidents, too. Little stuff, though, never anything major like today's ridiculous rap beefs where someone winds up getting shot. Nobody was trying to be a gangster. We handled our riffs by throwing rhymes and attitude.

OVER THE NEXT several years, our stars continued to brighten. The standard we'd set with our first album was quickly surpassed by our next couple of efforts. *King of Rock*, which I consider a decent album though not a great one, cemented our marriage of rock and hip-hop. Our next album, *Raising Hell*, is considered by many to be the greatest rap album of all time. Containing hits like "It's Tricky," "My

Adidas," "Peter Piper," and our cover of Aerosmith's "Walk This Way," *Raising Hell* was the first hip-hop album to go triple platinum. Three million records sold for a hip-hop album in 1986? That was considered impossible. There were people who'd never bought a rap album before and haven't bought one since, but they bought *Raising Hell*. Our fourth album was *Tougher Than Leather*. It wasn't considered the equivalent of its predecessor, but we knew going in that it was going to be nearly impossible to outdo *Raising Hell*. I mean, *Tougher Than Leather* wasn't our worst effort, but it certainly wasn't what the previous three were. It marked the first time since we'd stepped onto the scene that our momentum slowed noticeably.

Then came our fifth album, *Back from Hell*. Up till then, our ride to the top had had plenty of bumps, but the trajectory had always been upward. By the time we started recording *Back from Hell*, I don't even know that I could even call us much of a group anymore. In putting the album together we were never in the studio at the same time. Run wasn't anywhere to be found. He had decided that family was more important. Jay was getting his. He was hanging out with all of these new guys. He was Onyx's producer. He was hanging with musicians, going out of state on DJ gigs.

I, on the other hand, wasn't doing much that was productive. I was pissy drunk all the time, slurring and stumbling around just to deal with my personal unhappiness, especially as Run-DMC's shine faded. I knew the haze of success couldn't last and that I would soon have to confront my true feelings about the falseness of my life.

I was fucking up. Run was fucking up. Jay was fucking up. There was no career powwow. There were no staff meetings to address our fuckups. There was no Russell calling us and saying, "Here's what we're going to do." He and his fellow record executive Lyor Cohen were worrying about building Def Jam, not the group.

Yet even though we were on the decline, in Russell's eyes, and in the eyes of the executives at Profile, we were viewed as being on the same level as Bon Jovi. We were that big at one point. But we didn't ever establish ourselves at a Bon Jovi level. It's like we were in a raft. Bon Jovi is floating, but all these new motherfuckers got speedboats coming around. We had become complacent. We should've made a move. We should have gone to a new label and regrouped.

You know what hip-hop group did it? The Beasties. They went to Russell and Def Jam's co-owner Rick Rubin and said, "Let us go." It freed them up to keep evolving musically. It allowed them to be themselves and grow naturally at the same time. The Beastie Boys rhymed the same way on all their records, with the same deliveries and all of that, but they changed feeling. They always kept, not necessarily the same look, but a sound that was uniquely theirs. They always kept true to who they were.

In contrast, during the period when we recorded *Back from Hell*, we were all over the place. Our time had nothing to do with doing dope songs. We were all separated. I felt like I was isolated in an artistic jail and that they wouldn't let me out to bring what I needed to the group.

Many of my years in Run-DMC were spent feeling like an unneeded third wheel. After our first album, my role in the group steadily diminished. I still recorded, but Run and Jay had little use for any of my creative ideas. Whenever I would suggest we try recording a song a certain way or use a certain beat or add certain lyrics, they would more often scoff at or ignore me rather than embrace my recommendations. I resented how they made me feel, but I was also too afraid of rocking the boat to speak up. I didn't want them to think I was weak or that I craved their approval, so I kept quiet.

What we failed to see was that our music worked only when Run and D. and Jay did it. It didn't work when just Run and Jay did it. It didn't work when Jay and the producer Baby D did it. It worked only when Jay, Run, and D. did it.

It's like the classic story of the pro football player who gets the big contract, the endorsement deals and shit, and then forgets that playing football is what got him where he is. As a band, we had lost our truth. We tried to do music that wasn't authentic. I felt like it was a gimmick. I know it didn't feel right. *Back from Hell* was a commercial disappointment. It was in line with the other shortcomings that had been building since I'd let my brother talk me into selling my beloved comics to get his turntables. I hadn't finished college. I was also drinking and smoking too much weed. Rather than face my issues early on, I continued my destructive behavior.

When we started out, we practiced all the time, every night. By *Back from Hell*, even before, we weren't doing that no more. Me and Run weren't even talking unless we were on the road or if we had a show or an interview. We had grown totally apart. Even the process of preparing for the album wasn't a collective effort. We were just components of something that now came together only when it was time to do music. Even if you think *Tougher Than Leather* was a good album, if you'd seen us by 1989, 1990, it would have been obvious to you that we ain't have no business making another album together. We should have known that with all the new groups out there, staying on top wasn't going to be easy. And we should've never even attempted to make *Back from Hell*.

We should've done what the Beatles did. See, the Beatles broke up at the height of their shit. We could've stayed a group. Come together just for shows, you know what I'm saying? I do know if we were older rockers, we would've understood that. We were only together for a short period before we blew up, so our rise to fame was a little different. We didn't have this old band thing. We didn't build the bottom-up following. We just came and shocked the world. So we could've continued to tour because people loved our older music. But as far as recording new material, we really should've let it go then. Because by the 1990s, it was even more dope-ass dudes coming, Redman, K-Solo, the Wu-Tang Clan. Tupac was around the corner. Nas and AZ. Jay-Z. Those motherfuckers was bubbling. Despite the brief resurgence we enjoyed in '93 with *Down with the King*, that decade belonged to a new crop of MCs.

After a six-year hiatus, in 1999 the label and the group had started planning another record. Did I want to be part of it? No. But did I understand why Jay and Run wanted to keep recording? Of course. Despite my melancholy moods, I respected their drive. I didn't expect them to use my desire to steer clear of them as an excuse not to work. We were professionals, men with families to feed, and they made a professional decision to keep it moving. It wasn't the call to continue working that bothered me. It was their inability to see things from my perspective, though, that drove me nuts.

To my way of thinking, why call me for a record or a video appearance if I can't participate as an MC and if you don't want me as a songwriter? Run and Russell didn't want my input on the songs and on the production of the record. To me, the whole effort was a waste of my time. But they kept at it.

I wasn't buying that line of bullshit, though.

"Hold up," I replied. "My voice is gone, I can't rhyme, and you want my name on an album?"

I was tired of disappointing our fans with lackluster efforts. I was tired of having my name associated with music that I didn't have a major hand in, that I didn't like, and that I no longer wanted to be associated with. And it wasn't just about me. I could've taken the check, OK, but what about our audience? What about our legacy? What about what the brand had come to represent in recent years, the brand that Russell was so ready to promote? My voice was completely gone, so what rationale would make you think, *Yo, put out this record and because it says "Run-DMC" people will want it*? It was like these guys hadn't learned any of the lessons from what we went through with *Back from Hell*.

I told Russell point-blank: "Put a fuckin' Run record out. Here's your chance. Do whatever you want. But leave me the fuck alone."

I didn't abandon the group. We released our last album, *Crown Royal*, in 2001. I couldn't contribute like I normally would have, but I made a couple of appearances. I think I wrote only one original verse on the entire project, as Run still wasn't interested in my contributions as a collaborator. I didn't care. I just wanted to get the project wrapped up and move on. To this day, I really don't know any of the songs on it, not even the ones where I actually showed up. Although the group's name is on it, *Crown Royal* isn't really a Run-DMC album. It's a Run album.

Of course, that didn't stop Run and the label executives from trying to use me when they thought it would be to their advantage, the way they did when they wanted me in that LA video shoot for "Rock Show."

As I said before, I showed up, mostly as a favor to Jay. But I stood in the video like a robot. I didn't participate in the jumping around and posing shit the others wound up doing in the video. I didn't even like the record. It was bull.

Jay asked me later why I just stood there.

I said, "Jay, I can't rhyme no more. Does it really make sense for me to run around and pretend I'm part of this record?"

He shook his head to say no. Jay knew I was right.

Run-DMC, one of the sources of both stability and pain in my life, was done.

A little more than a year later, a gunshot stole Jam Master Jay's life, effectively ending the group anyway. With Jay gone, I knew that the label and Russell would have even less inclination to want me around. We had attended this school together called Run-DMC and, finally, we had graduated. I wished Run well, but I had no inclination to see him anymore. Even before Jay's death, Run was going around telling people how I couldn't rap anymore because of my vocal condition, so he was going to have to move on without me. With Jay dead, the chasm between me and Run widened even further. I last saw him at Jay's funeral. It would be more than seven years before we would speak again—and even then it would be for mostly professional reasons. But fuck it, I was long past the point where I expected anything resembling friendship from Run. I knew our friendship had hardened into a business relationship years earlier, and now that Run-DMC business was officially over, I had no expectations that he would be in my life at all. I was good with that. It wasn't as though I felt Run did something to me. He didn't. We had moved in our separate directions.

FIVE

IDENTITY CRISIS

A FAMILY SECRET REVEALED

I n 2000, I was searching for a new project to work on. With my voice shot and Run-DMC essentially defunct, I decided the time had come for me to pull my life story together. I set about some personal research. My first stop, of course, was to my mother, Bannah McDaniels. Since she had been there from my conception, I assumed there was no better place to start finding out more about myself than her.

On September 22, I gave her a call to get some of the basic details about my birth—what time I was born and where, how much I weighed, the difficulty of the delivery, and the like. I imagined she'd rattle off whatever she could recall, and I would circle back to her later to pick up any additional details she might have left out. It was a call that wouldn't last longer than a few minutes. I thought it'd be an easy story to tell. After all, if anybody I knew had had a stable, normal upbringing, it was me.

My parents, who had come up to New York separately from the South as younger people, were solid, hardworking role models for me and my brother, Alfred. My mother and father got along great as a couple and, as parents, always seemed to be able to handle their sons without losing their emotional balance. Even after I became a rap star, my parents never tripped on my fame or my money. They wouldn't even let me move them into a new house until Run-DMC was on like our third or fourth album. They were calm, practical people who went with an even keel about almost everything. They were generous without spoiling us. They weren't cheap, but they were sensible. I learned a lot from watching how they handled themselves.

My father, Byford McDaniels, had come from Jacksonville, Florida, to New York at sixteen years old, working several odd jobs before signing up for the Merchant Marine. He learned engineering in the Merchant Marine. After serving in the Korean War, he returned to New York City and spent the next forty years as a boiler-repair specialist for the city's Metropolitan Transportation Authority.

My father was an upright man, but even though I went to Catholic schools for most of my life, he and my mother weren't overly religious or anything. They had a practical form of morality that demanded that they work hard, raise decent kids, treat friends and neighbors with respect, and carry themselves with dignity.

This is the story I tell that, to me, sums up my father: Way back when Run-DMC was first starting out, we did this show in Brooklyn at a club that was owned by a notorious mob boss. Just before we were supposed to go on, I was in the dressing room with Run and Jay, and two infamous gangsters, when the owner's dad walked in. These guys looked like they'd walked straight off the set of *The Godfather* or something, all scowling and beady-eyed. One of them walks up to us and goes, "Which one is Mac's son?"

I'm thinking, *Who the fuck is this guy and how does he know my father?* I didn't want to admit who I was. Jay and Run quickly stabbed their fingers in my direction and said, "That's Darryl right there!" *Gee, thanks, fellas.*

The guys walked up to me and immediately started shaking my hand real hard. "Oh my God, Darryl, we just want to tell you that your father is the best man we have ever met. A great guy! If he ever needs *anything*, all he has to do is let us know." The emphasis they put on the word "anything" made my blood run a little chilly and my jaw drop.

My dad wasn't a gangster or a criminal by any means. He was just a hard-toiling, blue-collar transplant from Florida. But he knew how to quietly command respect from anyone, usually because he also knew how to show them respect as well.

My mother, Bannah McDaniels, injected much of the fun and humor into our family life. She was a beautiful woman, a Claire Huxtable type, who had come up to New York from Olar, South Carolina. She loved to cook and host parties. Every family event turned into a jam with her around, whether it was a Christmas Day dinner or a birthday get-together for me or my brother, Alfred. She was a registered nurse and a hard worker just like my pops. Every day, it seemed, the two of them battled to see who was going to get out the door first to grind the hardest. They both worked my entire life, even after I started getting money. My mother's first job was in Queens, at a hospital. Later, she wound up working in this other health facility in Rockaway called Haven Manor. When she got the job at Haven Manor, she was set.

My parents were strict, but they were cool as hell, especially when they were younger. They sent me to the best schools they could afford. During the weekends, my parents were never home at the same time due to their work schedules. Weekends, my father might be home all day Saturday, then at eight in the morning on Sunday he was on his way to work. They made sure that our whole family took a trip every year. They would take that one week and say, "Oh, we gonna drive to Canada." Taking a vacation was a big deal because most people in our neighborhood couldn't afford to take them.

Their relationship was openly loving, warm, and close. I remember that from when we were little up until I was like fifteen, we always had babysitters, because my parents would go to the movies to see *The Exorcist* or *Shaft* or a Fred Williamson film. They went to see all the blaxploitation movies.

My family and I lived on 197th Street and Hollis. Ours was the quiet part of the neighborhood, whereas the area past 200th Street was known to be wilder. Two Hundredth Street was sort of the dividing line in Hollis, the street that separated the more serene part of the neighborhood from the places where the thugs hung out. Some of my friends lived above 200th—including Run and Jay—but as a kid, I mostly stuck to my part of the neighborhood.

Our neighborhood was as practical as my parents. In the early 1970s, Hollis, Queens, was a predominantly black, blue-collar neighborhood whose streets were a testament to the ambition and work ethic of our parents. Rows of small, neat homes stretched along each block. Small businesses, from bodegas to shoe stores to dress shops, thrived. Like many places in New York, Hollis had its challenges— drug abuse, random crime, occasional outbursts of serious violence—but for the most part, it was still a place where children could play and families could grow.

It was all so . . . normal. So when I rang up my mom

and tossed out my handful of basic "what, when, where" questions, I expected her to recite the facts as easily as she could recollect the alphabet or her favorite recipe. After about a ten-second pause, she began running down what she remembered: "Let's see, you were a morning baby. You were born at nine thirty in the morning."

There was a short pause, then she continued. "You were a big baby. You weighed eight pounds, ten ounces, and you were born in New York Hospital."

I grinned a bit, scribbled the information onto a little pad, then rushed off the phone with a quick "Thanks, Ma. Love you."

A few minutes after I hung up, my phone rang. My caller ID showed that it was my mother. I assumed my mom was doing what she often did after we talked—calling back to make sure everything was going OK with me. I picked up the receiver and soon realized that this was not one of her usual return phone calls.

"Hi. Darryl, it's us," my mother began.

"We have something else to tell you," she said, the pace of her speech quickening as she talked. "You were a month old when we brought you home. Darryl, you're adopted . . . and we love you very much."

My body froze. Meanwhile, my mind raced at one hundred miles per hour. My mother's words echoed through my head as if she'd shouted into the Grand Canyon: "You're adopted . . . you're adopted . . . you're adopted . . ." As I stood there holding the phone in stunned silence, it felt like long hours were passing by.

My mother tried to break my trance, her voice soaked with worry. "Are you still there? Darryl?"

More silence.

Then my father, sensing my mother's panic, interjected. "Darryl," he said slowly. "Are you OK?"

OK? Hell no, I wasn't OK. My mind was playing back the early years of my life in reverse, flipping back through from college to high school to my days in the schoolyard at Saint Pascal's. I struggled to dig up any fragment of memory that might help me make sense of what my mother had just told me.

Finally, I mumbled a reply. "Just . . . just give me a minute to let this soak in."

We got off the phone shortly after that. When my parents called the next day, my mind was still reeling. With my father on one line and my mom on another, my mother started to lay out bits and pieces of my past, at least as far as she knew them. "We think that your mother's name is Bernada. She was really young when she had you. We think she was sixteen, and we think that you might be Dominican."

The surreal nature of it all slowly began to set in. I felt like I had just been thrust into the Queens, New York, version of Arnold Schwarzenegger's movie *Total Recall*. I immediately remembered the film's tagline: "What would you do if someone stole your mind?"

The flashbacks continued, growing more vivid with each memory of my childhood. My upbringing was one that many kids would envy, filled with loving and attentive parents, family cookouts, unforgettable Christmases, and raucous Thanksgivings and birthdays. I thought about our family trips, house parties, even hanging out in the patio furniture we had in our yard. I remembered the Electra 225 my dad used to drive, the basketball hoop where me and Butter and Dexter and Run would play.

The memories shifted to those strange, random fragments that I had been searching for, which began to fall into place. I recalled when I was five and a kid named Oscar came to live with us for a few months. I remember the day his mother came and took him away and I never saw him again. Shortly thereafter, another little girl came home with my parents. She cried so hard and so long that nobody was able to sleep for almost the entire night. I finally fell asleep around two thirty in the morning and, when I woke up the next morning, the girl was gone. Hindsight kicked in. *Foster kids!* They were foster kids that my mother and father were taking care of. I probably started off as one of those kids.

I thought back to being outside with my friends at seven and eight years old and how, when they got upset with me, my friends would taunt: "Darryl, you're adopted, you don't even look like anybody in your family." "Darryl, why don't you look like anybody in your family?" "You're not theirs." "That's not your brother." "That's not your father." I ignored them, chalking their teasing up to jealousy over the idyllic life my family enjoyed.

I recalled going through puberty and how, between ages fifteen and seventeen, when my arms started filling out and I shot up in height, I'd glance over at my mother and father and think, *What's wrong with this picture?* My father looked like Cliff Huxtable. My mother looked like Claire Huxtable. Alfred, my brother, looked like Eddie Murphy. *How did I come out looking like this?* I would wonder sometimes, before quickly waving off such thinking. I *had* to be their child. They were all I had ever known. Any thoughts of me not belonging to the McDaniels family were always quickly discarded.

Suddenly, a voice crashed through my reverie. "Darryl? Darryl, are you there?" It was my father.

Barely able to speak I murmured, "Uh-huh, uh-huh." I wasn't there, though.

"We'll help you find her," my father assured me.

He and my mother asked again if I was OK.

"Uh-huh, I'm cool," I lied. "Bye . . . I love you."

I hung up the phone and collapsed into the nearest chair. The flashbacks continued to run, flickering in my head like an old-time newsreel. I remembered the first time I brought my wife, Zuri, to Long Island to meet my parents. "Why don't you look like anybody in the pictures?" she'd asked. "Why aren't there more pictures of you? Where are your little baby pictures? Where are the baby pictures people get when they first come out of the hospital wrapped in a blanket?" I didn't know the answers, but it wasn't enough to make me doubt who had brought me into this world.

Zuri would even ask my mother, "Who does Darryl look like in the family?"

My mother used to fib and say, "He looks like his grandfather."

In looking at pictures of my grandfather, I would always say to myself, *The only thing I have in common with this man is height*. It still wasn't enough to make me question my identity.

In the fantasy worlds I used to construct, my identity had always been fluid. As a little kid, I could transform instantly into any of the countless superheroes whose adventures filled the pages of the comic books I collected. Later, as a teenager cultivating my love for hip-hop, I had taken on numerous aliases. Easy Dee. The Devastating Mic Controller. Years later, I was the King of Rock. Meanwhile, my lyrics were also ferocious declarations of who I always knew myself to really be. I was the "son of Byford, brother of Al." I was the kid who, after high school, "went straight to college." Everything in my life had been built upon the firm bedrock foundation of my life as Darryl McDaniels.

And now that foundation had been rocked.

THERE WAS NO underestimating the impact of my parents' news on me. For most of us, family is our first social crucible, the first place we form our values and opinions and perceptions of ourselves and the world. Family is where we learn that we are good and special and that we belong. Certainly that had been the case for me. It was outside the family where I felt bad about myself.

I started to wonder why my birth mother had decided to give me up for adoption. Hadn't she loved me? Didn't she think I was worth her making an effort to keep me? Wasn't I good enough? Did she miss me? Here I was, a world-famous musician with millions of admirers, and yet I was consumed with a deep sadness at the prospect that the woman who was supposed to have been the most important person in my life, my mom, hadn't wanted me.

I was messed up badly for the next several months. The strain of losing my voice and the decline of Run-DMC had been hard enough. And now, abruptly, I was told that my parents weren't really the people who'd brought me into this world. Not long after I found out, I began drinking heavily again.

My relapse into alcohol abuse came as a range of emotions roiled inside me. I bounced from anger to deep sadness to confusion to fear. I was outraged that my parents, as well as other relatives who knew the truth, had kept such a secret from me for so long. I was heartbroken at the prospect that I'd never know the woman who had brought me into this world. I was curious, too, but more than anything, I was terrified at the possibility that since I suddenly didn't know who I was, I was actually nobody at all.

When I reached out to a few of those around me for emotional support, I got mixed reactions. Thankfully, Jay, for one, was very supportive. He was a family man, too, so he knew how devastated I was at the realization that I wasn't an actual McDaniels after all—but he was one of the first people to remind me that Byford and Bannah loved me no matter what. He reminded me just how much my adoptive parents had sacrificed to ensure that I'd had such a nice upbringing. He couldn't truly fathom my pain, but at least Jay tried to comfort me.

However, Run was far less sympathetic. When I told him about my parents' revelation, about the confusion and pain that had followed, he looked at me as if I'd just read him the weather report. His face was a complete blank. In fact, the only way I even knew he had heard me was by what came out of his mouth next.

"Bannah and Byford are your parents, D. Suck it up. Let the other shit go!"

And then he walked off.

I'd just gotten the most earth-shattering news of my life. I figured I might be able to expect just a sliver of compassion or, at the very least, lurid interest. Nothing. Run made clear that he couldn't give less than a fuck about me or my problems. And with that, I was determined to cut him out of my life forever. When I changed phone numbers, I didn't bother to tell him. I stopped talking to him about anything personal at all. I talked only about business with him, when Erik couldn't do it for me.

Not surprisingly, my most abundant source of support came from the same people who'd dropped that bomb on me to begin with—my mom and dad. For long weeks after their revelation, they called and visited to make sure I was OK. They encouraged me to satisfy my curiosity about my biological mom by seeking her out, if that's what I wanted. They were genuinely sorry at the shock and pain their news had caused. I learned that they'd never really planned to tell me, but they were willing to give me the room to work out my feelings. I wasn't mad at them.

It wasn't easy for everyone, though. When I started my search for my birth mother in 2004, my brother, Alfred, was taking care of my adoptive mom, and he suddenly became very protective of her. My father was gone, she was physically ill, and so, like a good son, Alfred wanted to make sure that whatever anxieties I was carrying didn't fall onto her. When I began filming the search for my birth mom with the music network VH1, Alfred turned down requests to be interviewed. He wouldn't let them talk to my mother, either. His attitude toward me changed. His attitude was, "Hold on, man. *You're* adopted. Why're you bringing this shit to her? Whatever you're going through, don't put that on *my* mother. Keep that shit over there to yourself."

I understand now. He was the one taking care of her. He had a home. I had an apartment. He worked at Con Edison; I was traveling all the time. It was tough on him. He didn't need money. He needed me to be able to take her for a week, go on a walk with her, spend time shopping. But I was caught up in my own shit, and he didn't really get it or have time for it.

It hurt me then. It put a strain on my relationship with Alfred for a long time—and Alfred and I have always been cool. We don't talk a lot, but we always call on the holidays, birthdays, other special occasions. And we know it's all love. But after that adoption program in '04, my brother and I didn't say a single word to each other for about a year.

We got through it, though—thanks to our wives. One day, I had to go over to his house to take care of some paperwork. My wife was with me, and when I got there, his wife was there, too. They were both tired of us not talking and they made that clear, like, "Look, this is getting old. You two motherfuckers need to talk, and we're not leaving until you do." And that's what we did. We worked it out. Since then, we've talked about my adoption, my birth mother. He's asked me questions about her: "How is she?" "What does she look like?" Alfred cares, and I understand that better than ever.

That's just how it is with family, those ups and downs. On one hand, nobody knows you as intimately. Rarely does anyone know the worst about you—your weaknesses, your insecurities—the way family does. As a result, not many people have the power to hurt you as deeply.

But on the other hand, not many people can comfort and assure you like family, either. Our mothers, fathers, brothers, cousins, wives, husbands—they can offer a reservoir of hope and perseverance. They aren't perfect, of course. They don't have all the answers, but they care enough to try to hold you up when you're down. That's why it's so dangerous to turn from their embrace when you're depressed or suicidal or even just mildly upset. Family is an integral part of your support system. You run *to* family's embrace, not away from it. If your biological family doesn't provide that comfort, establish one that does through a network of friends and health professionals. It's a necessary source of strength.

Whenever I contemplated suicide, even though I never told anyone I wanted to kill myself, my mind often turned to my wife or my mom or my dad. When I tumbled off the wagon with a thud in 2000, my family refused to stand idly by while I drowned in liquor. My wife stayed on me about getting help. My closest friends hounded me, too.

When you're depressed, it's easy to look past the most natural support system you have. It's easy to judge your value by those blind to your worth rather than by those who cherish you the most. But that's also one of the biggest mistakes you can make.

Men are taught to offer help, but too often we don't know how to receive it, not even from the most natural places. When I was struggling with the news of my adoption, there were times when I turned away from everyone. There were days when I chose to suffer quietly rather than have my wife or mom offer me soothing words.

There's a certain narcissism with the pain men go through. We think that nobody else can possibly fathom it, that no other person has ever hurt the way we do. We're wrong, of course, but it's hard to have that kind of perspective when you're depressed or scared or convinced of your worthlessness.

In time, though, my family and friends did get through to me. Along with the encouragement from my wife and parents, one of the biggest boosts I got was from an adoption support group I joined at the urging of my friend Sheila Jaffe, the famed casting director, who is an adoptee herself.

When I found out I was adopted, I felt for the longest time like I was alone. But at the first meeting of the support group, I quickly realized just how not alone I was. Suddenly I was part of a community filled with a diverse group of people, from doctors and lawyers to blue-collar laborers and Hollywood bigwigs. All of them were talking—sometimes calmly, oftentimes with nearly violent anger—about adoption, foster care, and how unfair the laws were that pertained to these issues. Although I didn't know shit about the political issues at the time and wasn't quite sure how the support group was going to help me with my personal issues, I returned every month to hear more. Each time I went, I spoke only sparingly, preferring to mostly sit quietly and listen to other people's stories. Sometimes, I'd join in the laughter—we joked a lot, just to keep from crying at times. But when the conversations got more heated, I'd close up.

After a while, someone in the group decided to call me out: "Darryl, you're handling this with a lot of human amusement and I like your lighthearted approach—but aren't you mad?" The question shocked me.

"Mad about what?" I shot back.

A few others spoke up: "Mad that your mother and father and everybody you knew all *lied* to you for all those years."

I gave what I thought at the time was the most honest answer I could muster. "No, they didn't affect me," I said. "They lied to me for a good reason, and even though they knew, I turned out all right and it helped me."

I was content with that answer as I gave it. But over the following few days, I started to reflect, and, slowly, a different type of sentiment started to surface. My thinking began to change. *They did lie to me! Everything was a front.* I began to consider the possibility that I was avoiding some hard questions about my circumstances.

At those meetings, the other support-group members continually encouraged me to think about launching a search for my biological mom: "You can go online, Darryl." "You can hire a private eye." "Now that we've got Facebook, you can check there." "You can go do your own research."

At first, I was hesitant. Part of me wanted to know, but I was also nervous about opening that door. There was no telling what was really behind it. The support group kept insisting I try. At each meeting, they'd poke at me: "Don't you really want to know?" And every time I said no, their efforts redoubled. Then, at one particular support-group gathering, an adoptee said something that sealed the deal for me. "Your life is like a book," she said. "And you don't ever start a book at chapter two. You start from the very beginning." It made more sense than she could've known. Her words stayed with me. Eventually I gave in and admitted that I did want to know, that, in many ways, I *needed* to know.

One of the reasons I came around was because I wanted to get a better understanding of my health history. When you find out you're adopted, it changes your whole truth about you physically. For all the love and life lessons that Byford and Bannah McDaniels had imparted to me, my DNA had come from elsewhere. If I had any predispositions to diseases or disabilities, I probably needed to know. Did my mom have history of heart disease? Had my father's family been prone to cancer? As much as nurture had shaped me and my future, nature still had a big hand in who I was.

My curiosity extended far beyond a desire to know more about my medical history. For me, as with many adoptees, I was far more concerned with the issue of why I had been put up for adoption. Whatever the circumstances I'd been born into, I felt like I had a human right to know what they were. If my mother had left me a cab, I had a right to know that. If my father had been the worst rapist/killer on the face of the earth, it was my right to know.

I could see from my support group how not knowing about a part of their lives had hurt so many people. I remember a guy from Australia who would talk, and it seemed that every time he opened his mouth, the pain just came rushing out. There was another lady who had been orphaned during the Korean War and was devastated to her core by the reality that she'd never know who her biological parents were. The more I contemplated looking for my birth mother, the more I began to believe that my search might actually help someone other than myself.

If I was going to look for my birth mom, I knew I had to stop drinking first. I wanted to be as whole as I could. I wanted my birth mom to see me at my best. I entered into rehab, which helped me more than I could have ever imagined. When I left rehab, I hadn't just dealt with my drinking. I'd dealt with the reasons why I was drinking. I left clean, sober, and sane.

I was ready to meet my biological mother.

IT TOOK ME several months, but with help from a private eye, I was able to track down my biological mom. It was harder than I thought, because the system is set up to discourage adoptees from looking for their birth parents. The people who run the system don't want adoptees unexpectedly showing up in their birth mothers' lives. Maybe the mom is married and never told her husband or her other children that she had given up a child. A revelation like that could ruin a marriage. Maybe the parents don't want to deal with the pain that comes with being reminded of the child they put up for adoption. The myth is that adoption laws are set up to "protect" adoptees. The truth is, adoption laws protect everybody except the adoptee. In all but nine states—Alabama, Alaska, Delaware, Illinois, Kansas, Maine, New Hampshire, Oregon, and Tennessee—adoptees are not allowed to get a copy of their original birth certificate.

I was persistent. After numerous frustrating encounters with the New York State adoption system, I finally traced my birth mom to an apartment on Staten Island. I learned that her name is Berncenia Lovelace. The private eye managed to get her address and phone number. After much trepidation—the first time I went to her door to meet her I actually ran away before she could answer—I finally found the courage to introduce myself by phone.

I was nervous as hell when I made that call. My voice almost cracked when she picked up the phone and said hello. I started slowly: "Um, hello, Ms. Lovelace . . . I have reason to believe . . . that I might be your son. I'm adopted and I'm looking for my mother. I think that you might be she."

After I finished, all she said was, "When were you born?"

"May 31, 1964."

"Wow, that's possible." And then she asked, "What would you like to do?"

"I would like to meet you."

"OK, when?"

"Like, right now?"

She wasn't ready right then. A whole lot was happening really fast, for both of us. She asked if she could call me back the following Saturday with a decision. I was cool with that.

I was stunned to find her, but disappointed that I had been the only one actively looking. I could imagine what it was like for her, to be at home minding her business and suddenly getting a call out of nowhere from a grown man claiming to be her long-lost son. I wouldn't have been surprised if she'd never called me again.

Before I could call her on Saturday, she called me the Friday before. "You know, I've been thinking about all of this," she explained, "but I don't want to wait to ask these questions until tomorrow when I see you." She started to toss out a few questions: "Are you married?" "Do you have kids?"

Then she said, "What do you do?"

I told her I was in the music business and that I was into rap.

"What's the name of your group?"

"Run-DMC . . ."

At first, she got really quiet. I'm thinking, *I just ruined it because she don't like hip-hop.* But then the pitch of her voice got really high: "Oh. My. God."

"What? You don't like rap?"

"No, I *hate* rap music. . . . But I *love* Run-DMC."

I was relieved. We chuckled about that for a second, talked a bit more, and then she told me, "OK, I'm all right with meeting you—but first, I have to go tell my kids."

My brothers, her sons, were understandably cautious when she broke the news to them. They weren't so much concerned about her past. I found out later that my sister had actually known our mother had had a baby who she'd given up. They were mostly concerned about making sure our mother was safe when she met me. Their thing was,

"Yo, Ma, when you meet him, you better do it in Starbucks or some other public place, because there are psychos out there."

Ultimately, we decided we'd meet her at her apartment: me; my wife, Zuri; and our son, D'Son. When the apartment door opened, it was the first time in my life that I'd seen somebody who looked exactly like me. Once I saw her, it really sank in. Until then, the whole journey had almost seemed like a dream, like make-believe, like it was somebody else's story and I was just an actor in a TV show. When that door opened, something inside me said, *Oh shit, D. You're really fucking adopted!*

When I walked into her apartment, I was struck almost immediately by some of the similarities. In my mom's apartment, she had the same exact Buddhist statue that I have. She had the same books that I read. On my arm, I've got my wife's name, Zuri, which means "beautiful" in Swahili. On my birth mother's arm, she has the tattoo in Spanish for "beautiful."

I met my two brothers and it got even crazier. My brother Mark, who's three years older than me, looks like me. Same height. Same build. He wears glasses. He's got a goatee. He draws.

His whole life, he said: "1984, 'Rock Box' comes out. 'Mark, Mark, come here! You look exactly like that guy, DMC, he could be your brother!' '85, 'Mark, Mark, come here! That guy DMC could be . . .' '86, 'Yo, Mark, Mark, come here!' '87, 'Mark, Mark, Mark!' '88, it was like this: 'Yo, Mark, Mark—'" It got to the point where he became fed up with motherfuckers calling him every time a Run-DMC video came on. "Yeah, I *know*. I'm fucking DMC's brother. I'm tired of that bullshit!"

My brother Damon, who is three years younger than me, he's a physical trainer and heavy into exercise like I am. My sister, Jayydiah, she has obsessive-compulsive disorder, just like me.

Eventually, as we sat there talking, we got around to what had brought me to Berncenia Lovelace's doorstep in the first place. "Do you want to know why I gave you up?" she asked.

I'm thinking, *Yeah, that's an understatement.*

She just looked at me and said, "To give you a chance."

What had happened was, her family had been living in Hamilton Heights, up in Harlem, and then her father had moved his family to Staten Island because it was less hectic. Harlem and the Bronx, back in the day, were ill. But though her father had moved the family to Staten Island, her boyfriend was still up in Harlem. Her dad was like, "You don't go back to see that guy!" At eighteen years old, she had come home pregnant with my brother Mark. Three years later, she came home pregnant with me. Mark was raised in the house with her and her parents and the rest of the kids. There was no room for me. There was no money for me.

My biological mom waited to have me and then decided to give me up for adoption. She didn't give me up because she wanted to or because she didn't love me. "I did it," she repeated, "so you could actually have a chance in life."

When she said that, all I could think was, *Well, lady, you gave me one* hell *of a chance!*

MY MOTHER AND I remained in contact and have grown closer over the years. In her own way, she, too, has been a source of strength for me. She loves me just as much as my adoptive parents do and, almost from the time we met, has been as emotionally available to me and my family as she is to the children she raised. She's a sounding board for my ideas and concerns and triumphs. She's a grandmother to D'Son. She's a friend to my wife. With both my adoptive parents now dead, my birth mom has become as much a mother figure to me as Bannah McDaniels was—and I know that's just the way my adoptive mom would have wanted it. In fact, Bannah made this clear to me years ago, after I found myself in what I feared was a holiday dilemma involving her and my birth mom.

It was the first Christmas since I'd found Berncenia, and I wasn't sure which mom I was supposed to spend the holiday with. I was really excited about getting to know my birth mom, but I also needed my adoptive mom to be secure in the fact that I still loved her, too. How could I spend time with one without hurting or offending the other? As usual, I wanted to please everyone—Bannah, Berncenia, Alfred, my biological siblings—and I had become stressed at the realization that I couldn't. It got so bad that I actually went to my counselor to frantically explain my confusion and indecisiveness.

I had begun to think that my childhood wasn't as rich as that of other kids because I was adopted and had been a foster kid. So I'm blubbering to the therapist about "being a foster kid" this and "being a foster kid" that. But the therapist checked me on that real fast.

"What makes you so different?" she said.

"Because, you know, I was a foster kid."

She said, "Hold up, wait. You eat and sleep just like everybody else?"

I was like, "Yeah."

"You got people around here that love you like everybody else, right? You was able to do stuff like every other little kid? So what makes you different?"

I was like, "Because I was—"

She said, "A foster kid, I know. Darryl, being a foster child doesn't make you a different *person* than anybody else. It just makes your *situation* different." She made me look up the word "foster" in the dictionary. As it related to foster child, it just mentioned a temporary placement for a child, a stopover you made in hopes of finding a permanent home. The only thing that made my circumstances different, she went on, was that my process of nurturing had been different. I was still a kid like any other. I had been conceived like any other kid. I had been birthed like any other kid. Once I was taken in, I had been raised like any other kid. I had nothing to be humiliated about.

"Christmas is coming and I've got my birth mother, but I've also got my mom-mom," I told her. "I don't know how to handle this. I've got to go see my birth mother. But I also don't want my adoptive mother . . ."

She cut me off with a wave of her hand and offered the simplest advice: "First of all, calm down. Second of all, what is it that you want to do?"

I told her that I really just wanted to stay home with my wife and son because that's really what I enjoy most on holidays.

She smiled at me and said, "Well then, just stay home with your wife and son."

At first I gave her this crazy look. "Huh? It's that easy?"

"It's that easy," she said. And then she told me this: "Your birth mother has her own life. And your adoptive mother and father have their own lives. Give them both a call at Christmas—and you stay home."

I did just that. And it was fine. Nobody was hurt. Everybody got on with their lives.

I had learned a valuable lesson. At its best, family doesn't fan anxiety or fear. Family gives you the space and the encouragement to do what makes you happy, and it finds contentment, not resentment, in that. Family wants to see you whole.

Bannah made this clear to me not long after that same Christmas. Even though the holiday had gone fine, I was still nagged by worries that she might be feeling overlooked. So that Monday comes, and I take my mom out to lunch. On Tuesday, I went and got her and took her to breakfast. Wednesday, I came and took her to dinner. The next day, I took her to breakfast again. On Friday, I took her to lunch. I remember her sipping soup as we were sitting there, at this Chinese restaurant near her house. I was staring at her.

Then, without even looking up, she says to me, "Darryl?"

"Uh-huh," I go.

"I don't want to see your ass no more."

"Huh?"

"I know what you're doing, and I want you to know that I understand. But I don't want to see you no more. Don't come get me again. You don't have to do this. I get it."

I had to laugh. She knew I was feeling guilty about having found my birth mom and knew I wanted to assure her that I still loved her just as much as I always had. But she understood. She knew there was room for both of them, in my heart and in my life. After the secret had finally been aired, I felt bad for her and my father, because I understood the pressure they had been under and how terrible they must've felt about seeing me go through my struggles over being adopted. I thought I had something to prove to them, but I didn't. Neither they nor my birth mother ever wanted me to feel bad over what had happened. Once I realized that, it was like the weight that everyone else had been forced to carry was now lifted off me, too.

I learned to think of it this way: The word "adoption" starts with "A." Birth starts with "B." My A mom, my adoptive mother, was who I'd known most of my life, so she had come first to me. But my B mom, my birth mother, she was an essential part of that motherhood thing, too. Without her, I wouldn't be in this world at all. I didn't have to choose. I didn't have to prioritize. I could just love them both and be loved. It was a wonderful revelation.

I carry that with me whenever I speak to foster kids and adoptees. The way it eventually came out even rhymed, although that was totally unintentional. I tell them, "If we can remove the guilt and the shame, we'll remove the pain." Remove the guilt and the shame of the birth mother who was forced to give up a kid. Remove the guilt and the shame of the adoptive family that conceals the truth. Only one person has the power to remove the guilt and the shame: the adoptee. I realized that I had no decision in the transaction that moved me from one home to another. But

I'm the one with the power to fix it. Not no law. Not no prayer. Not no religion.

It goes back to the same lessons I learned in rehab. Whether it's a work decision, whether it's family decision, or whether it's a relationship decision, if it's messed up, I'm the one who has the power to heal it.

SIX

BALANCING ACT

FROM A STRONG
BODY COMES A
SOUND MIND

SIX

A blast of body heat and the clatter of iron greeted me as I walked through the door of the gym for the first time. All around, toned women in spandex and hulking dudes in tank-top shirts were grunting their way through push-ups and bench presses and carefully choreographed aerobic routines. Trainers barked instructions at sweaty middle-aged men struggling through gut-busting ab regimens. Fitness freaks with sculpted frames preened in the mirrors mounted throughout the place. They looked to be in the prime of their lives.

Me, I was there trying to avoid dying.

It was 1991, and, after a nearly two-month stay in the hospital for the pancreatitis that had resulted from my alcohol abuse, I was following up on my doctor's directions to find something better to do than drink cases of Olde

English 800. The warning he'd issued—"You drink, you die"—rang in my head in concert with the barbells clattering nearby. After two months in the hospital, I had decided that not only was I going to stop abusing alcohol, but I was also going to try to replace my bad habits with some good ones. I resolved to start exercising regularly.

But now, gawking at the towering stacks of iron plates and intimidating exercise machines and massive bodies running effortlessly through endless calisthenics, I just prayed I could get through the next hour without passing out. You know the saying that what doesn't kill you makes you stronger? Well, right then, I was hoping that what was supposed to make me stronger didn't kill my ass.

Working out hurt like hell the first few days, but I stuck with it. Gradually, my routines intensified. I began lifting and running longer. Before I realized it, exercise had become a fundamental part of my lifestyle.

Aside from sending me to the hospital with pancreatitis, getting regularly drunk and high had also created a chemical imbalance in my body and, surely, my brain. I was using the substances to fight depression or loneliness or suicidal thoughts. It didn't work, but the gym helped. I was sweating out the toxins from the alcohol, which meant my body was beginning to correct some of the imbalances that I had created with my abusive behavior. The gym high was actually better than the drink high. The gym high made me feel energetic and a little like I could do anything. At times while lifting weights, I had insights into my true personality. The thoughts were fleeting and came usually as I moved on to another machine. It was a good space for me. The gym offered structure and routine. It also allowed me to feel safe. I could set simple goals, such as one hundred push-ups. And when I accomplished them, I felt good. The gym was an immediate high.

Addressing my diet and getting into the gym meant that I was ready for a physical change. But I was still an emotional wreck. After all, my drinking had started as a substitute for the confidence I lacked when I was sober. It had become my way of repressing my feelings whenever I was hurt or pissed off. But I didn't understand that in 1991. All I knew at that time was that I had nearly destroyed myself with malt liquor.

Throughout my teens and early twenties, I'd weighed barely more than 200 pounds. As a result of years of ceaseless drinking, I'd ballooned to more than 240 pounds. My stomach was paunchy. My face was puffy. My eyes were always red.

I may have loved the buzz I got from downing bottle after bottle of beer, but I was displeased by the physical side effects. In looking to better my body, I came to realize that physical exercise was essential to the fitness of my mind and soul, too.

Going through depression for me was a sedentary endeavor. When I was at my lowest point emotionally, I didn't want to do much but sit on my butt and feel lousy. The weed made me sometimes overeat or turn to binging on comfort food like ice cream or cookies. And the alcohol was rich in calories. The alcohol also diminished my motivation. My vision was clouded to the point where I was convinced there was no future for me.

I sat around many days, at home or in my car or in the studio, sulking and wallowing in self-pity and simmering in unspoken rage. I drank while wondering, *How do other people do it? How do they move through life so effortlessly and free of feeling stuck?* The only part of my life I maintained was trying to create music, but even when I made it to the studio, I'd often show up too intoxicated to be any good. I remember when we were making *Back from Hell*, Jay put my ass out of the studio a few times because I was slurring my lyrics. I couldn't get my act together enough to do even the one thing I still had a passion for, which was rap. I was continually focused on my interpersonal strife and emotional turmoil.

When I started lifting weights and doing cardio, I found another, more productive outlet for some of my emotional pain. I realized I could sweat out some of the anger rather than attempt to numb it. Taking care of my body gave me something else to think about. In the beginning, I had to force myself to go to the gym every day. I would tell myself, *This is the one thing that I have to do today.* It was tough. Every morning, the same dialogue in my head.

Come on, Darryl, you can do it. Maybe I won't go today, but I'll go tomorrow. No, you have to do it. Just this one thing. I started to believe that if every day I could make myself do something, it would help me get past my depression. Help me get out of my own head.

I started developing goals for my time at the gym. I grew determined to lift more, to run farther, and to work out longer than I did the day before. These goals gave me something positive to strive for and at times displaced negative thoughts. The endorphins produced by my body when exercising affected my mood. Some people get a real high from working out, which can stick with them for a whole day. For some, especially if they are dealing with depression, it offers relief in the short term. But I believed that exercise could put me on the right track toward healing.

My consistency in going to the gym affected my life immensely. Along the way, I found that exercise gave me more energy during my shows. When I was a drinker, it seemed like it took forever to get through performances. Without the alcohol, it was as if I could rip through shows faster even than I did back in the early 1980s.

I'm in my fifties now, and I'm probably in better shape than half the younger musicians I meet. In fact, I use age as a motivator. I'm a grizzled veteran in what is supposedly a young man's game. But I say all the time, "Real MCs don't get old." I shouldn't have to age out of music any more than you should be forced out of law or architecture or retail sales or whatever it is. I'm not about to let anyone tell me that I can't still enjoy being an MC.

The only way I can keep up physically is to do the same thing I've tried to do to keep pace lyrically: prepare. When we were nineteen and twenty years old, Run and Jay and I could zip through entire shows as if we were jogging to the corner bodega. Even when I was drunk off my ass, it was easy to bring the requisite energy to our stage show. Being older now doesn't mean I'm not as good as I was then. It does mean, though, that I've got to take better care of my body in order to stay at the top of my game as a performer.

Exercise and diet are important. Of course, because I have an addictive personality, I crave exercise these days much the same way I once craved drugs or alcohol. Working out has become my new vice and, in some ways, I struggle with this, too, as a result of my psychological makeup. For instance, when I was going through rehab, I was restricted to an hour for my workouts, meaning I was forced to choose between doing cardio exercises or lifting weights—when I had become accustomed to being able to do both. It killed me to have to choose!

Fortunately, my devotion to exercise has yielded benefits, both to my body and my artistry. One of the excuses I use when I get obsessive about exercise is that it is not only good for my body and mind—it's great for my creativity. In one workout session, I can have a whole song written and completed, without writing down one word.

I'm not suggesting you be obsessive about exercise, only that you be a good steward of your body. Unfortunately, most of us aren't. Studies show that about 35 percent of adults in the United States are obese. More than 39 percent of adults ages forty to fifty-nine are obese, while 30 percent of adults ages twenty to thirty-nine suffer from obesity.

In impoverished neighborhoods, obesity and other health issues are an ever-bigger problem. Hypertension and diabetes result from social conditions that leave many of us trapped in poverty and unable to access quality food or health care. And then there's the pressure, the trauma even, of living in a nation where we're overwhelmed by violence. People in poorer neighborhoods face the worst treatment by the police. They're jailed more often for lesser or equal offenses than those in richer neighborhoods. The inequality creates a level of stress that can wreck havoc on the mind. Many try to numb themselves from the stress with food.

As ardently as I'd embraced working out and eating right in the early 1990s, I relapsed back into hard drinking in 2000—even though I knew exactly how much harm I'd do to myself and to my family. I had been living cleanly until then, but the depression that came with finding out I was adopted was more than I was prepared to cope with. Even though I had stopped drinking and had improved my physical condition, I hadn't yet begun repair on my tattered emotions. I hadn't shored up my coping mechanisms.

I drifted away from the regimen that had treated me so well during the nine years I was sober. I hurt my body. I gave in, again, to the inertia of depression.

It took me four years to pull out of that tailspin. Therapy and family pulled me through. Since then, I have maintained my physical fitness regimen.

I know a little about being busy, and exercise helps me maintain my professional schedule and emotional equilibrium. Even now, in the latter part of my music career, it seems like I'm always climbing onto some red-eye flight west or some international flight overseas. If I'm not on a plane, I'm often being squeezed by an itinerary loaded with in-store appearances, TV interviews, studio sessions, and production meetings.

I remind myself: *This is your body.* Caring for my body is as much an act of self-love as is embracing the people and things that bring me joy. It's essential to my overall wellness, allowing me to dwell on positive, self-affirming thoughts.

Whether I'm just landing in a new town or getting ready to play my final show of a tour, I always find time to exercise. Even when I'm tired or stressed, I figure out how to make my way to the gym. Sometimes I can find a Gold's Gym, where I'm a member, in one of the cities I'm visiting. Other times, I'll have to make do with the fitness center of my hotel. I'll lift for an hour, do another forty-five minutes to an hour of cardio, and usually leave feeling like a new man. If there are no weights or treadmills around, I'll do calisthenics to stay in shape. I don't make excuses for not working out.

As serious as I am about my physical health, though, I'm just as serious about balancing that by staying mentally and emotionally fit. Learning to care for your mental health is a lot like developing a workout routine: You go on a diet, dropping things that are not healthy for you. You start working out, dealing with the baggage you carry. And just as with exercise, you've got to figure out what works for you. It's all on the individual; it's all on the dedication that you put into it; then once you get a result, it's all about being strong enough to maintain it.

I needed therapy even more than I needed to exercise, and I'd probably needed it for much of my life because of all the pain and resentment I had bottled up inside. Being drunk all the time had deadened the pain enough for me to act like it wasn't a big deal. Alcohol was my camouflage, but behind that facade were feelings that had turned toxic long ago. They had also gotten out of control. I used to find myself seething with rage or tumbling into depression, and I wouldn't know why or what to do. I had spent so many years neglecting my feelings and lying to myself that I had no idea why I felt what I felt or how I could handle it without poisoning myself with guilt and rage and sadness. Even when I had gotten to the point where I didn't want to kill myself, I still needed to learn how not to hurt myself.

That's where counseling came into play. After rehab, I began taking more intimate steps in my mental health recovery. As part of the VH1 Rock Doc that was documenting my quest to find my biological mom, the show's producers had hooked me up with a therapist, figuring I might need someone to talk to if the experience got to be too tough. When they first suggested it, I was cool with the idea, but, in my mind, I saw it as just another part of the show, not as something that would have any lasting impact on me personally. After all, I'd worked all that out in alcohol rehab, right?

Wrong.

I had three sessions with the guy, all of them filmed for the show. I'd go to his office on the Upper West Side, sit in his waiting room in this big chair, with a bunch of *New Yorker* magazines scattered around. The first session, he comes out the door with a patient, and the patient just looked awful, a white guy probably in his late thirties. He just looked like a zombie. When I looked at him he just stared past me. I said, "Hi," but he didn't say a word to me. It wasn't exactly a ringing endorsement of my therapist— but I didn't let that deter me.

And I'm glad it didn't. For those three sessions, we got into discussions about how I felt about my mother, how she was still my mom even though I didn't come from her, all that. We discussed my frustrations with the adoption system, my fears about being accepted by my birth mom.

At first it didn't feel like it was me at the center of this TV program. Sure, I was doing this Rock Doc search, but it didn't feel like it was about me. It just felt like I was doing this because I'm adopted. I'm doing this for somebody else that's adopted. That was the first session. By the last therapy session with the guy, though, we had gotten to the point where I was telling him my fears about how my adoptive parents really felt about me. Did they love me? How could they love me and wait so long to reveal something like me being adopted? Were they ashamed? But you know the biggest revelation from those sessions? I realized just how much more I really needed therapy.

That's the funny thing about opening yourself up to mental and emotional healing: you often don't know just how much you need help until you start to get a little. With your body, the signs that you need to improve are outward and obvious. But mental baggage doesn't show like that, so it's easier to overlook—until it becomes unbearable. Going to those first few therapy sessions made me realize I couldn't look past my psychic unhealthiness anymore.

As helpful as those counseling sessions were, though, they were still just for the Rock Doc that VH1 was producing. After the program aired, I paid out of my own pocket to start seeing my own therapist, a woman named Dr. Wendy Freund. I met Wendy through the New York Foundling, one of the oldest and largest child services agencies in New York. Wendy serves as a therapist in the foster-care system.

Her job there is to prep children who are about to be placed with a family, to try to help them adjust. If I were to compare my mental health therapy to physical exercise, then Wendy was my personal trainer.

She doesn't look imposing. She's a short lady, with a short haircut kind of like Halle Berry's. She's got a small frame, but she's got that spunk. She kind of reminds me of Estelle Getty from the television show *The Golden Girls*. She's like the cool grandmother, elderly but still swift and spry.

Despite her looks, though, Wendy was thorough and unflinching in her observations. She didn't lay out solutions to the issues I was wrestling with as much as she let me discover them for myself. She allowed me to understand that I had the answers to my problems. A lot of times, it didn't even seem like our conversations were getting deep. I'd walk into her office at New York Foundling, and she'd open up by asking me simply, "How are you feeling today? What happened?" From there, I'd start to let it all pour out—the questions, the fears, the heartache.

Wendy helped me understand that I had the power to heal—myself as well as others around me. I could heal myself by getting to the root of my problems, by addressing my issues honestly, and by acting in an honest and forthright manner with others. A lot of my anxieties and depression were rooted in my unwillingness to put myself first in certain situations, in choosing to go along with other people's agendas instead. She helped me understand that there is nothing wrong with being selfish in certain ways, because otherwise you can find yourself doing things that make you unhappy. Now if there's something I really don't want to do—if I know that I'm going to leave that thing feeling bad—I just don't do it. I say no. If someone asks me to an event, for example, and I just don't like the people or the atmosphere, I don't go. In the past, I would have. Not anymore. Why should I be uncomfortable or vexed just to satisfy someone else? There's nothing wrong with being considerate—but you don't owe it to anybody to be in uncomfortable or hurtful situations.

I learned I could heal my family and friends through forgiveness and understanding. My adoptive mother and father didn't have to carry the guilt of keeping my adoption a secret for so many years, not if I assured them that I loved them and was OK. Same for my cousins and brother and everyone else who had worked so hard to not tell little Darryl the truth about where he'd come from. Meanwhile, on the flip side, my birth mom didn't have to carry any guilt about giving me up for adoption as long as I made sure she understood that I wasn't angry or hurt, just thankful to finally get to know her.

All that power was within me. I just had to find ways to tap it. And the best way was to be truthful, about myself, my feelings, and my intentions. I learned to start getting back to the things I enjoy, whether comic books or my light rock or reading. Before I was in Run-DMC, I read all the time. I had all kinds of books, novels, comics. As a kid, my imagination was everything, and reading was the fuel for that imagination. I realized how I'd gotten away from a lot of that once I'd gotten into hip-hop. Once I was in the group, it was about recording and tours and concerts and writing rhymes. I don't think I really started reading again until I started in rehab. When I was there, I was reading Deepak Chopra and a bunch of metaphysical stuff. But until then, I'd left my love of reading behind—and in so doing, I'd abandoned a big part of myself.

Wendy helped me get back to this by assuring me that it was OK not to care about what people thought of me. It was like, "So what if those motherfuckers don't like it?"— but in a grandmotherly way. Not only was it OK to be myself, she assured me, it was also critical to my health.

In trying to get away from myself, I had fallen into drinking and smoking. The drugs and alcohol allowed me to play a part, to function in the outside world. To fit in. But what the fuck did I need to fit in for? Why wasn't who I was good enough?

Wendy helped me see something that I share with kids to this day: The most powerful thing that you can do is be true to yourself. With pride, say that you love comic books. With pride, say, "I love to draw!" I was just telling this to students at a middle school I spoke at. I said, if you play the violin, be proud that you can play the violin, and say it with the same enthusiasm that another guy says, "I got guns and I got girls and I got new sneakers." Say, "I play the violin," and if you say it with the same enthusiasm you'll shut the other guys down. They will bow to you, because they will look at you and think, *That's powerful.* If you can play the piano, if you're a dude that wears a tutu and you got to go dance with Misty Copeland and do ballet, you say, "Yes, I dance with the ballet and I wear a tutu and I travel to Russia and I'm dancing at Carnegie Hall!"

I said to those students, "Look what I did." I said, "I came out and said, *I'm DMC. In the place to be/I go to Saint John's University, and since kindergarten . . .*" I could have said, "DMC takes what some people might say is the most corny thing—going to college—and makes it the most powerful thing." If you draw, if you dance, if you like poetry, if you like spoken word, whatever, if you like polka dots—use who you are, who you *really* are, as a positive. That's your superpower.

Wendy helped me see the need to ground myself that way again. Grounding yourself in your truth and embracing who you are also makes it easier for you to deal with problems you encounter with others. Used to be, if someone did something that pissed me off, it made me wonder what was wrong with me. I used to question myself and what I'd done, what kind of person I was. Now? If someone does something to piss me off, that's on that person. His or her actions have nothing to do with who I am or what I'm about. They don't define me in any way.

I don't see Wendy as often as I used to—the last time we spoke was just before I got back onstage with Run for the first time since Jay's death—but I'm still working to put into practice everything she counseled me on. Still, I committed myself to the hard work just as I'd dedicated myself to getting and staying in shape years ago. Healing mentally was no more instantaneous than cutting all that beer fat from my body. It has taken years of toil. On both counts, though, the results have been immensely satisfying.

SEVEN

LOSING A LITTLE OF MYSELF

COPING WITH VIOLENCE AND DEATH

I didn't believe the news when I heard it.

It was late October 2002, the night before Halloween, and I was packing to travel to Washington, DC, for a halftime performance at an NBA game. A television was blaring in a corner of my bedroom. The voice of the channel 5 anchorman was part of the background noise as I piled jeans and T-shirts into my overnight bag. My wife was nearby, chatting with me casually between occasional glances at the TV screen.

Then the talking head said something that made both of us jerk to attention: ". . . again, Jam Master Jay, part of the legendary rap group Run-DMC, has reportedly been killed."

I rolled my eyes and waved my hand dismissively at the screen. I wasn't buying it. This wasn't even the first time Jay had reportedly been killed. During the *Raising Hell* tour in the late 1980s, a rumor had circulated that Jay had died while out on the road. In 1990, news reports had claimed the same thing after Jay had been shot in the leg and wounded outside a club during the Christmas holiday. I knew better, though. Jay had turned out to be fine then, and I was certain he was OK now. I was looking forward to seeing him in DC the next day, and knew we'd laugh about this silly mistake. I kept packing.

An hour later, though, on the channel 9 eleven o'clock newscast, I heard a reporter repeat the bulletin that had come across at ten p.m.: "Jam Master Jay, DJ for famed rap group Run-DMC, has been fatally shot at his studio tonight . . ." This time, I paid closer attention, as the reporter's tone seemed much graver, more certain. I still wasn't worried, though. I was thinking about how we'd have to spend the upcoming days shooting down rumors of Jay's demise.

I quickly turned to channel 11—and they had footage of cops outside the studio and emergency medical personnel bringing out a body bag. *Nah*, I'm thinking. *They've got this all wrong.* Obviously, something bad had happened at Jay's studio, but that couldn't be him zipped up in that black bag. Whoever it was, it wasn't my DJ.

The phone rang. It was my manager's daughter—and she was crying hard. "They killed Jay," she sobbed into the phone.

Zuri and I jumped into our car and jetted to Jay's studio, which wasn't far from the old neighborhood in Hollis. When we arrived, I got out of the car and walked to the curb. I saw Chuck D. from Public Enemy and the former MTV personality Ed Lover a few feet away, crying like babies. The police walked over—the precinct was right across the street from the studio!—and asked me fifty million questions.

It was during their questioning that it hit me: one of my closest friends had been murdered. Memories of Jay came flooding back—our childhoods in Queens, our first time recording together, our first out-of-town trip, all the nights we'd spent staying up after shows to drink and smoke and laugh and dream together. Jay had stood by me when I lost my voice. Jay had been warm and supportive and a positive influence in my life.

Jay was my business partner, my friend, my brother. Now, in the flash of a gun muzzle, he was gone, and no one had any idea why. Growing up in Queens, I knew of guys who'd been killed, but I'd never lost anyone this close to me this violently, this randomly. I clutched my wife's hand and started crying right there outside the studio.

A week before Jay's death, Run had left the Aerosmith tour, forcing our entire group to come off the road prematurely. After threatening to come apart for years, Run-DMC finally unraveled. Run wanted out. I was mired in alcoholism. Now Jam Master Jay was dead. If there were doubts before, things were painfully clear this October night: Run-DMC was done.

A week after Jay was shot, Russell and Run called a press conference to announce that Run-DMC was "retired." They never consulted with me or anyone else about the decision. I didn't even get word about it until they called me on the morning the press conference was scheduled to take place and asked me to come. It took me totally by surprise. I showed up mainly out of respect for Jay.

To make matters worse, the media put Jay's financial business out in the street, mentioning how he owed a $500,000 tax debt. I remember Chuck D. and everyone who was close to the group being really upset about that. I'm not denying that it was a matter of public record because of the investigation, but why bring it up at this press conference? And really, why wait only a week to call a press conference at all? Was our "retirement" really such big news at that point, or was someone just trying to capitalize on a publicity opportunity? Everyone was still buggin' about the fact that our friend had been killed. We could've waited before getting up in front of the media to say some stuff like that. Emotions were still too raw, the hurt still too fresh, to be grandstanding.

I know that *my* family and friends were all wounded, in addition to being confused and angry. I remember my dad being totally perplexed: "Jay? Why would *anybody* want to kill Jay?" he asked over and over, his face contorted as much by confusion as by grief.

The only answer I had—for anything at that point—was to turn up a bottle. I was so fucked up that I couldn't even mourn properly. I was caught up in my own issues. Losing Jay just forced me deeper into those negative feelings. For weeks, I slammed glass after glass of whiskey and wondered just how much worse life could get.

A month after Jay died, my father, Byford McDaniels, passed away from liver cancer.

There was an ironic inversion to his death and Jay's. Whereas Jay had died while working, my father died precisely because he wasn't working. Years before the cancer claimed his life, my dad had been diagnosed with diabetes, and we'd always worried that that would be the end of him. But the diabetes never stopped him from staying active, and he continued to find odd jobs, whether they were for friends or family, to keep himself busy. Well after he'd retired from the MTA, and long after I'd moved my parents out of Hollis to Freeport, Long Island, in 1986, my dad could be found mowing someone's lawn or fixing a car or repairing something inside a home. He would go visit friends just so he could fix things. Almost every week, he would leave the house and call me or Alfred and ask, "Is there anything that I can do?" When my wife was pregnant, he would come to the house just so he could drive her to her doctors' appointments. He was always buying tools and gadgets advertised on those late-night infomercials and then looking for reasons to use them. Every morning, he would wake up looking for something to do. Even after he'd been diagnosed with liver cancer, my father did whatever he could to stay active.

In 1999, my parents moved from their house in Long Island and went down south, to an area around Columbia, South Carolina, where my mother and her family were from. My dad hated it because he didn't have anything to keep him busy. In New York, he had felt useful, lively. But after my parents moved to the South, my dad didn't have anything to do except sit around. He didn't have any activities or odd jobs to keep his mind off his illnesses or to serve as his own brand of physical therapy. He would try. Occasionally, he'd drive from South Carolina to Jacksonville, Florida, his hometown, to meet up with friends or family. But even then, other than making the actual drive, he wound up doing very little. The inactivity took as much a toll on his spirit as the cancer did on his body. A few years after he went back down south, my dad was dead.

I never got a chance to say good-bye to my dad, as the cancer, once it really took hold, consumed him faster than any of us expected. When I found out he had passed, the news, combined with the lingering grief over Jay, left me feeling almost paralyzed for days. I couldn't talk. Couldn't think. All I could muster the energy to do was cry while getting as drunk as I possibly could. I remember the night before his funeral I got so drunk that I passed out. When I came to, I went to the service, mourned my dad, and fell even harder into alcohol abuse.

My fall back into alcoholism was aggressive. Until I'd contracted pancreatitis, drinking had been fun. Sure, I might've used it as an escape from some of the anxieties and professional problems I was faced with, but my life was going great back then by comparison. Now, in a matter of two months, I'd lost one of my closest friends and my father. Two of the most supportive pillars in my life were gone.

ALL LOSS HURTS—but violence gives an even darker dimension to loss. In the nearly fifteen years since Jay was shot to death, I still don't have the words to adequately describe what his passing did to me, what it still does to me. To call the loss of Jay devastating seems almost like an understatement. When I learned about his death, it took a chunk of my soul.

I know that I'm not alone in dealing with that kind of trauma. Violence has become more prevalent all over the world. Many believe that the violence promoted in some hip-hop music is one contributor. Our music was fun. Hip-hop started out as party music to get the dance floor rocking. It was followed by socially and politically conscious rap, then gangster rap.

Witnessing violence is life-changing.

Violence shadows us daily, be it as an actual act, a direct threat, or simply the allusion to it that we experience. Fans and artists in hip-hop are, unfortunately, denizens of some of the most violence-plagued communities in the United States. Homicide remains the leading cause of death for black boys and young men. According to federal statistics, slightly more than 50 percent of the deaths of black males aged fifteen to nineteen are the result of homicide—mostly by gunshot. Similarly, homicide is the cause of nearly half of all deaths of black men aged twenty to thirty-four. We experience way too much violence in our neighborhoods. Our streets are lined with makeshift memorials of candles, RIP graffiti. Many of us have lost friends to violence. Mourning has become a dominant pastime. The prospect of violent death scares us. Yet many of us adopt a "ready to die" mind-set. Death, such people figure, is inevitable, and it's likely to come violently and suddenly. So why not live like there's no tomorrow? And why not hide behind a callous disregard for others?

I still grapple with the death of Jay because of how unexpected it was. I never got a chance to say good-bye. I have held on to a piece of him by rocking Jay's signature "JMJ" belt whenever I perform.

JAY WAS CLOSE to my heart and also at the very center of what Run-DMC was all about. Run-DMC would never have been the group we became without our Jam Master Jay. In many ways, Jason Mizell was Run-DMC long before me and Run ever were. Even before we started rapping together, much of what Run-DMC would be known for was defined by Jay.

Jay had grown up in Hollis, same as me and Run, but Jay had grown up a lot faster than we did. He was up on all the fashions before us, and not just the kid stuff, but that grown-man stuff. When we were still wearing whatever our parents bought us in the teen section of the store, Jay had the lambskin coats and the Playboy shoes and the Pierre Cardin shirts and pants. He had a kid first. He was the first to lose his dad, to have to become the man of his house. Jay was grown, yo.

He probably wouldn't have ever had reason to mess with nerds like me and Run if it weren't for hip-hop. Back when we first started, the DJ was all-important. In fact, you could argue that the DJ was at least as important, if not more so, than the rappers who stood in front of him. While hip-hop is thought of today as a purely lyrical exercise, it was in fact dominated by the DJs back then. If we were going to be successful, we needed someone to back us up on the turntables.

Originally, Run had two DJs in mind, but neither could take the gig. One of the guys had already started his own DJ collective and wanted to see that through. The second guy took a job at the post office, which seemed like it had a whole lot brighter future than spinning records at the time.

We remembered this other DJ, who was, at least to us, the next best thing to the other two. He might've been something of a wild guy, always with the Hollis crew whenever we'd see them down on Forty-Second Street in Manhattan doing their thing, but we also knew from the parties around our neighborhood that there weren't many DJs better than the kid who back then called himself "Jazzy Jay."

We went looking for Jay, and eventually found him hanging out up on Hollis Avenue. Run went up to him and was like, "Yo, me and Darryl made a record. We need a DJ. You want to be our DJ? We've got this gig coming up in November. We're going to get paid."

Once Run mentioned the money, Jay was down almost immediately: "Hold up. You mean I'm going to get paid to do what I do in the park for free? Hell yeah! That's dope!"

From the very beginning, Jay was more than just our DJ. Along with Larry Smith—the legendary producer who also created hits for Whodini, Slick Rick, and others—Jay was a coarchitect of our sound. Moreover, he was our look and feel, too. He gave us the style—the hats, the black leather, the laceless sneakers—that became our signature getup. From his pimped-out stroll to his fly gear to his hood-savvy attitude, Jay was the original mold for our overall aesthetic. When you saw our stoic grills staring out from album covers or movie posters, when you saw us sauntering from one end of the stage to the other, when you saw the tongues of those shell-toe Adidas rising up like tombstones, you were getting a glimpse of the vibe that Jay first brought to the group. Run and I weren't street guys. We were nerds from Queens. When I was barely more than a four-eyed comic geek and Run just the curly-haired little brother of an upstart party promoter, Jay was street for real.

I remember one night, we had a gig scheduled at the legendary Bronx club Disco Fever. We were returning to New York after being out on the West Coast for a minute. Getting together for sound check, we needed to pick up Jay. As we normally did, we pulled up in front of Jay's house. Russell and Larry were with me, and we knew that Jay was always running late. He was still inside. We had rocked Disco Fever the first time we played the venue and there was no way Jay was gonna miss a second. After a long wait, Jay finally walked outside. We all just stared.

He came out of the house with the four-speaker JVC boom box, the one with the two cassette-tape decks. He had on a pair of black Lee jeans that B-boys wore. He also had on a black leather blazer, a black sweatshirt, and his little gold chains. His Godfather hat was on his head. On his feet, he had on the Adidas we always wore—except, because he was running late, he hadn't had time to put the laces in his sneakers, so the tongues of his shoes were sticking straight up.

When Russell saw that, he knew. We all did. He spoke it before anyone else got a chance to. "That," said Russell, "is your wardrobe."

Me and Run saw how it fit. It was the consummate B-boy look of our era. It was cool. It was street. It was also still sharp enough to go onstage and shine. It was all Jay. It was perfect. Along with our leather blazers, our three-striped sweat suits, and, later, our gold ropes with the gold Adidas sneaker medallions, it would be the look that would define not just us but also an entire generation of our fans.

We were the first rappers to take the everyday look that kids rocked on the streets of New York to the major stages. Before us, most rappers wore disco outfits, skin-tight all-leather ensembles, or Native American head-dresses or some other type of costume. Armed with our wide-brimmed *Godfather*-style fedoras, our leather sport coats and stiff Lee jeans, and our unlaced Adidas shell-toe sneakers, we were the embodiment of a hardcore B-boy aesthetic. Most groups performed hip-hop shows looking as if they were ready for a night out at Studio 54, the famous celebrity discotheque. Not Run-DMC. We walked onstage like we'd just jumped off a subway car. Jay made us official.

Before Jay hooked up our look, I remember being in a dressing room with the Fearless Four, another legend-ary group. When they walked in, they came in like James Brown. They had their leather. They had their capes and their boots and their tassels. That was the thing with the Bronx; they were fly. And I'll never forget Mighty Mike C just looked at us and sort of shook his head.

"Y'all ain't even got a wardrobe," he said. "Y'all just got hats."

Those hats were all we needed.

Once we had mastered our routines, our look, and our basic sound, we went back into the studio and recorded "Hard Times," which was a social-commentary rap, like "The Message." We started touring the country shortly afterward, and more fans started to recognize me and Run. But when our group went out onstage, our fans would see three guys. That puzzled some people. *OK, I know DMC. And I know Run. But who's that guy on the turntables?*

I had already come up with an answer to that before the three of us even began performing together. As I've said, Jay's original name was Jazzy Jay (though sometimes he switched it up to Jazzy Jase). When we came out, there was already a DJ Jazzy Jay. I'm a connoisseur of hip-hop, which means biting is not allowed! So not long after Jay joined as our DJ, I told him that we'd get him a new name. "Don't worry, Jay, I got you," I said. "Give me a day or two."

I went home and thought, *All right, you've got the Grandmaster Flash. You've got the Grand Wizard Theodore. You've got the Grand Mixer DXT. You've got Afrika Bambaataa, DJ Red Alert. How do we get around this?*

The solution, of course, was right there at the foundation of hip-hop culture, resting amid those inspirational pillars I mentioned before, kung fu movies and comics. In comic books, you always had the *Invincible* Iron Man, the *Incredible* Hulk, the *Amazing* Spider-Man. I started thinking about Jay's role as both the party DJ and the guy who was the DJ for this group with these hits. That's when it hit me: "jam." The word "jam" has two meanings. The jam is the hit record that everyone likes. *"Yo, play that jam you played last night!"* It is also the party. *"Yo, that jam last night was crazy."* I said, "Jay's going to be the master of it all." Flash and them was just grand masters at the party. Jay's the master of that, too. And he's spinning records that are the jam.

When I caught up with Run and Jay later the next day, I said, "I got it." In front of Run and Jay, I told him: "You're Jam Master Jay." He loved it as soon as he heard it. "Yoooo!" That's all he kept saying. "Yo! Yooooo!!!" He realized instantly that it was unlike anybody else's name. Also, with Grandmaster Flash, Theodore, DJ Charlie Chase, and the Cold Crush Four, the DJ was always in front. When I created the name Jam Master Jay, I wrote a song to go with it:

> *J-A-Y are the letters of his name*
> *Cutting and scratching are the aspects of his game*
> *So check out the Master as he cuts these jams*

And look at us with the mics in our hands
Then take a count: 1–2–3
Jam Master Jay! Run! DMCeeeeee!

THROUGHOUT HIS CAREER, Jay represented a huge part of the heart and soul of Run-DMC. When we were at our best, it was because all three of us were grinding together, with Run steering us conceptually, me bringing the hardcore lyrics, and Jay doing the heavy lifting. Behind the turntables and the soundboard were Larry Smith and Rick Rubin. We were greater than the sum of our parts when we worked together.

Run might've just been a coworker after a while, but Jay remained not only one of my closest friends but also one of my great musical inspirations and one of the most motivating people I've ever been around. Jay could get me to do stuff when no one else could. He could bring out the best in me, even when I was pissy drunk and reeling in the studio.

Jay never turned his back on me. When I lost my voice, Jay suggested ways to keep me involved in the business. It was necessary for me to be a part of the marketing and promotion of Run-DMC. In addition to that, Jay encouraged me to ghostwrite for the many groups he was producing, as well as do some work in the studio. Even when *I* wasn't sure about whether I wanted to stay part of the group, Jay continued to assure me. "Yo, D., there will always be a place for you," he'd tell me over and over. "You will always have a way to feed your wife and family, no matter what happens." Jay never forgot that the three of us were supposed to be in this shit together.

The state of the band shortly before Jay's death was unfortunate. It adds to the pain. Run walked off on the group in the midst of a tour we were doing with Aerosmith and Kid Rock. Jay tried desperately to keep us on that tour. He tried to appeal to Run's sense of loyalty to the neighborhood, reminding him that many of the guys who were on tour with us were friends of ours whose entire livelihood rested with Run-DMC. Runny Ray, Erik, and Wendell "Hurricane" Fite—who was best known then as the Beastie Boys' DJ—were our people. They didn't have 401(k)s and severance packages waiting for them when we got off tour. We took care of them, and Jay never lost sight of that.

Run's words when we asked him to think about all the crew from Hollis who we'd be leaving ass-out by bolting from the tour? "They'd better learn to push mops. They are grown-ass men. They will figure it out." Nothing else Jay or Erik—who, at Run's insistence, had gotten us both more money and our own tour bus—could say would make Run change his mind. He wanted off the tour, and that was final. We'd all just have to try to live with it.

A few weeks later, the night before Halloween, as Aerosmith and Kid Rock played the Woodlands, in Texas, on the tour that we should've still been on, Jay was gunned down as he sat inside his recording studio. (No one has ever been arrested or charged for his murder.)

When Jay died, Run-DMC died with him. The world was a better place with Jay in it. It was a better place with my father in it. And, yeah, it's better with me in it, too. Losing those two important people in my life helped me see that. Jay loved life and was murdered, while, ironically, I was the one consumed with trying to kill myself. Suffering through the loss changed my views on what it means to be alive.

EIGHT

THE GREAT "I AM"

A SEARCH FOR SPIRITUAL CONTENTMENT

I grew up Catholic. I was an altar boy. I attended Catholic schools from elementary at Saint Pascal's to high school at Rice in Harlem. I knew all the priests and nuns in our parish. My family attended church fairly regularly, even though my parents weren't particularly zealous about religion at home. They were believers, but I don't think it made a big difference to them if everyone around them was. Unlike in some black households, Sundays didn't find our home filled with gospel or the raspy admonitions of a TV evangelist. I think my mother and father carried their religious beliefs in their hearts more than on their sleeves.

As I got older and started writing songs, I could see my Catholic upbringing diffused throughout my lyrics and song titles. Check the Run-DMC discography and you'll see album and song titles like "Raising Hell" and "Back from Hell." Peep my lyrics and you'll hear lines like, *"I cut the head off the devil and I throw it at you."* It's all from comic books and the Catholic church, man.

I wasn't all that concerned with issues of spirituality during much of my adult life. I was on the road having too wild a time to worry much about my eternal soul. I didn't really abandon any of the beliefs I'd been taught as much as I thought about them as nothing more than passing notions.

For most of my life, I've been more inclined to worry about things like how I'm treating people and how I'm presenting myself than about whether some god is watching me. One of the reasons why I think I never quit the group or just said "fuck you" to the people around me during even my worst days was because I was always worried about treating people like I wanted to be treated. Even if people weren't actually treating me how I wanted, I was an empathetic dude. A lot of musicians might think they're better than their fans or the roadies or the people who work the venues they perform. But I've never forgotten that I'm just some kid from Queens who got fortunate. It's tricky to keep one eye in front of you and one eye on where you've come from, but I've always believed that it is essential to have a certain moral balance. There's very little that separates people, and I have always tried to keep that squarely in mind. So I've never been quick to fight or even blow up at people. Maybe I was too self-conscious about who I was in the grand scheme of things—nobody, really—but I always tried to keep my karma or energy or conscience or whatever you want to call it clear and clean.

Back in the early nineties, Run and I found ourselves in something of a spiritual search. While I was kind of open to a lot of ideas and beliefs, Run had begun to get deeper into the Christian church. He was still doing little stuff like smoking weed at first, until he started to get really caught up in the church scene. He hadn't quite taken on the Rev. Run persona that he would eventually adopt, but Run—who had been drawn to ministers ever since we'd seen the street-corner preachers in Manhattan during our trips to the old porn theaters on Forty-Second Street—had begun to attend the Zoe Ministries church, which was run by a guy named Bishop E. Bernard Jordan. A lot of people say the bishop is just a hustler, one of those prosperity ministers always trying to scam people out of their money by using God and the Bible and whatnot. He was always on TV or making appearances somewhere, talking about money and his ministry. Run gravitated to him instantly. Since he was the front man for the group, he wanted to bring his new beliefs to the group, too. At first, Russell wasn't with that. He was fighting Run on the church tip and didn't want it on our next album at all.

Ultimately, Russell not only gave in, once he figured it worked for Run, but he also pushed it hard. I was disappointed in Russell. He wanted to take the G-O-D thing and apply it to the theme of the *Down with the King* album, because Run's in church and "Y'all got to change your look." Run cut his hair, got a bald head like me, and then started wearing crosses. "Y'all got to get a cross now." I remember sitting there and saying, "Hold on, this ain't got nothing to do with fuckin' Jesus!" The album title was supposed to be about being down with the King of Rock, the kings of rap. But they began trying to sell it as a reference to God. They pushed it on us, a gimmick. You look on the cover of *Down with the King* and not only do you see us in all black and with bald heads and me without my glasses, but you also see wooden crosses hanging from our necks.

Run was intense in his involvement with the church. Whatever Bishop Jordan's real intentions were, I think Run really bought into them. As we were making a comeback in 1993, he invited me to be part of his church, to heed the words of the bishop. When we'd go on the road or spend any time together ahead of interviews or studio sessions, he was constantly trying to convince me to come to his church. For a little while, I actually went. At first, I can't say I was completely drawn in, but I went. Then I joined. They pulled me in. "We need you to come all the time," they told me. They made me a deacon right away. Run had started as a deacon, too. Not long after that, Run started training to become an ordained minister. He became the Reverend Run, and I was supposed to be Deacon D. They were even using the *Down with the King* concept to promote their agenda. By 1995, I'm going all the time, not realizing this is some brainwashing.

I can say that now, looking back, but at the time, I was buying into a lot of what the Bishop was selling. After I'd spent so many years drunk, sobriety had now left me searching for advice and ideas about how to live my life, about how to keep making the sort of changes I felt I needed to get better. I can't say I didn't learn a lot, because I did. There was a lot of asking for money, but there were also times when I heard messages that were genuinely helpful. The church brought in all kinds of speakers, people from other churches and temples. Sometimes they would bring in motivational speakers instead of purely spiritual types. I remember Les Brown, that guy who was married to Gladys Knight at one time, showed up at the church. I was open to newness, and that made me open to a lot of the bishop's ideas. He would say, "All truths are parallel." Telling me that what was in the Quran was also in the Bible and in what Confucius said. "It's all in there."

I wasn't reading only what the Bishop gave me. I was studying all kinds of spirituality. I was trying to understand Jesus but also Siddhartha Gautama, Buddhism, as well as reading about fatalism and destiny and all of that. I was willing to learn. I think that's why I liked going. After years of drinking myself into a stupor, I was starved for clarity.

I also thought back to the existential crises I had gone through years before, in which I questioned my purpose and first began to acknowledge the void inside me. When I started to lose my voice, it was as if I had started to lose myself. I thought I was on earth only to be the "King of Rock" dude. When I feared that I couldn't be that guy anymore, I believed that my time had run its course. I had defined myself so narrowly that when I could no longer do the one thing I had always been great at, I began to believe it was time for me to end my life altogether.

I didn't drink myself to death. I didn't commit suicide. I didn't shoot up a crowd full of people and then turn the gun on myself. I was still there. Whatever power anybody wants to believe in—Buddha, Yahweh, the Holy One, the Almighty, whatever—had apparently decided that it wasn't my time.

Honestly, that whole brief Deacon D period was a dark, cloudy, uncomfortable period in my life when I felt worthless. I remember having to laugh when my man Runny Ray told me once, "Get that Deacon D bullshit out of here!" There were times when his voice was the only thing that I heard over and over. I wasn't high. I wasn't even drinking then. That whole Deacon D period was ugly for me on the inside. Life made no sense. That shit added to my depression.

No matter how I tried, Zoe Ministries wasn't the place I was going to find many answers. I may have gleaned some lessons and helpful information, but in the end, it was a hustle. The bishop. The guy was using me, using my money and my fame and celebrity to raise his profile. Given my condition, I was vulnerable to people like the bishop.

My wife always had her suspicions about the church. She never trusted the bishop. But because she was so supportive of me, she was cool about it at first and would attend with me. Then she saw that they were trying to take advantage of me. We were going on Sundays and that was cool, then they had a class another night. But if they had a session on Tuesday nights, Run would work it into the Run-DMC schedule. "Yo, me and Dee need to be home because we got to be at the bishop's." We used to have to work out flight tickets and whatever. It got to the point where it was stressful. My wife stopped coming, at first on Tuesdays and, after a while, completely. Tuesday night was the "deep" teaching, where it wasn't just Bible stuff. The bishop would tell you what books to read and this and that: "I'm going to teach you this. I'm a preacher of this Word here." He would also bring in some secular reading to make you feel like what he was saying wasn't just some religious craziness, that it was acceptable in intellectual circles. After Run and I started attending the Tuesday session, it wasn't long before they wanted to have sessions on Wednesdays, too. Then Thursdays. It grew into the bishop wanting us to fly with him to other churches, so he could get money from them, too. They were calling the house all the time, constantly trying to use me for this program or that lecture or this event. My wife soon asked me, "What are you doing?" It had become disrespectful to her when they started calling our house all the time. She was on the phone, yelling at them: "You got my husband on Sunday and Tuesday, now you calling my house? Oh, hell no!" That's when it felt cultish to both of us. They were trying to control our every move and our minds. They were trying to tell us what to do, how to spend our money, and who we could hang with.

I started looking at the bishop like, "Before, I was like a little child under your jurisdiction, hungry to learn and to be accepted. But now you have become completely intrusive." It didn't stop them. If I missed a Tuesday or a Wednesday, my phone would be ringing that same night.

"We just wanted to know what happened to you last night, Darryl."

My wife was angry every time they called. She started urging me not to go anymore. It was messing with my relationship with my significant other.

There were times when I wanted to curse them out— but I didn't do it. After a while, I just changed my number and slowly stopped going. When I finally got tired of it after the constant harassment, my wife's reaction was basically like, *What took you so long? I been saw that, the first day we went there.* One thing about women is, they're very emotional, so they tell you, "I never liked him the day I met him." Meanwhile, as a man, you think, *She's just hating*. Later you find out she was right.

GROWING UP CATHOLIC, I was always taught that we're weak and need to lean on God for everything, and that to do this, we need to go out and find God. Rehabilitation showed me that everything I needed I already had. In twelve-step rehabilitation programs like Alcoholics or Narcotics Anonymous, a big focus of the program is on getting addicts to turn themselves over to "God as we understand Him" or to a "Higher Power." That leads a lot of people to exit rehab mistakenly thinking that a Higher Power is going to be in some room with them like another person, rather than understanding that Divine power lies within. I realized that I *am* the Higher Power. It's my Higher Power, I have it, it's mine. The Higher Power and me are one and the same. God puts his power in us. I'm not looking for another being to come save me. The same way you say, "I am going to get a drink," you have to be strong and say, "I'm not going to get a drink." That's exercising your "Higher Power." After years of searching outside myself for answers—looking to weed and to drugs and to malt liquor—I now understand that once you find your true self, you find your Higher Power. You don't have to search for your God. Once you find yourself, God—your power— comes to you.

I was consumed with depression, but I wasn't going to get better just by sitting around wishing for a better life. I had to stand up, seek out counseling, perform self-examination, and challenge myself to do something to change my condition. It didn't matter what my religious beliefs were. What mattered was that I was trying to play an active role in my own salvation. Most major religions teach some variation of the idea that faith without work is dead. I can believe in a religious idea all I want, but I wouldn't change until I *did something* that allowed me to change.

I grew up in church praying to God in hopes that He would make my life better. But it was hard work—round-the-clock recording sessions, endless travel, paying dues on small, cramped stages in crappy little venues—that enabled me to have a successful music career. I had to put work in before anything positive happened. Religion had nothing do with it. And neither did some supernatural being out in space somewhere. I don't believe in that kind of god or that kind of religion. I think God is in us and wants to manifest itself as God without being labeled as separate from us.

I think people have to discover their own religion. The term "religion" means how you relate to yourself in your universe, something different. I read Deepak Chopra's books and I read the Bible four or five times from start to end and I went to Run's church—and none of that worked for me.

When the Bible didn't work, when Run's church didn't work, when Deepak Chopra didn't work, when metaphysics didn't work, Jack Daniel's and Jim Beam became my best friends, but it took my own revelation to realize this ain't working, either. The drinking thing was a false god. I was killing myself, committing suicide not knowing I was committing suicide. When the Bible didn't work, when Deepak Chopra didn't work, I had to write my own scripture and I had to ask, "How is this story going to turn out?'"

Well, I didn't know how it was going to turn out, but one thing was just not going to happen: I decided I was not going to die. It's crazy, but my life started turning for the better once I said I have the power to write my life, I have the power to create my story. I had to go through that whole process to realize that it all starts with the great "I Am."

NINE

FAMILY VALUE

DISCOVERING LOVE, FINDING FATHERHOOD

ike everybody, I've experienced a wide range of highs and lows in my life. I've enjoyed the euphoria of outstanding achievement. I've known fear and anger and most certainly depression. I've been humiliated and rejected.

However, romantic love I hadn't known until it came walking into my life in 1992, when I first met Zuri, the woman who would later become my wife.

Certainly, I'd always known the love of family. My mother and father, my brother, my cousins—they showered me with affection in their own ways. This love was another reason I had such a tough time dealing with the news that I was adopted. My family never treated me differently, never diminished me, never made me feel like I was in any way anything other than a McDaniels, born and bred. My older brother, Alfred, and I, though we didn't get to spend a lot of time together after he went into the army and I started making records, were always the sort of siblings who got along more than we fought. He was certainly my older brother, but we got along fine. He'd shoo me away from him and his friends when they'd be out on the block or in the basement playing music. We were a normal family in almost every way.

Even though I often talk about how depression inundated my life, you should know that, were it not for the love and support I received from my family during some of my dark periods, there are no guarantees I'd have made it. Good health, good friends, a strong sense of identity—these are all important. But my experiences in a loving, supportive home were invaluable. I knew men could be upright and loyal, because my dad showed that to my mother and my family. I knew women could be loving and beautiful and caring, because that's what my mother gave to her family and husband.

But romance? Even true self-love? Those were harder to come by for me.

Before I met Zuri, I'd carried crushes for a few girls. I remember I used to be in love with Runny Ray's beautiful sister. Other than a bout of puppy love here or there, most of my relationships with women were very transient, very temporary. I was on the road all the time. I was living in hotels and out of my suitcase. I was rarely in any one place for more than a few days other than New York City. Groupies made it easy for me to find entertainment without commitment.

In addition, as an alcoholic, I didn't make relationships a priority. Instead, I was somewhere trying to get to the bottom of a bottle. How can you focus on someone else when all your time is spent worrying about how to cater to your dysfunctional cravings? Jay and Run were just as busy as I was, but they had both gotten married and had families. I was so busy drinking that I never made time to develop anything long-term with a woman.

That's why I'm not all that surprised that Zuri and I got together soon after I'd ditched the Olde E during my struggle with pancreatitis. I was clear-eyed. I was in the best shape of my life, having lost weight and started the constant workouts that I continue to this day. I had cut my hair so I was bald and, at Zuri's insistence, I soon stopped wearing glasses. I was looking good, feeling good, and I was in a space where I could actually have a successful relationship if I wanted one. It's hard to claim to love someone else when you're constantly abusing yourself.

But with my wife, I knew almost as soon as I met her that I was ready to love that woman.

I was hanging out with Jay one day, walking along Broadway in Manhattan. He lived on Barrow Street in the city, so I'd always go over there to meet up with him and then we'd head to the studios together. We were working on *Down with the King* at the time, somewhere in 1992. We were doing some of the early sessions. I think we might've been waiting for Run to make one of his appearances that day, and we decided to walk to the deli. As we were making our way up the street, Jay spotted a group of young women he knew walking toward us. I think a few of them were R&B singers who had auditioned for him and a bunch of other producers who had done some studio work with Jay. He stopped to talk, but I wasn't paying a whole lot of attention. They were all cute girls or whatever, but I wasn't sweating them. Then I saw my wife-to-be in the crowd. I swear, as soon as I saw her, something in my head just immediately said, *That's my wife*.

Like I said, getting girls had never been a problem—c'mon, I was in the music industry—and New York City has always been full of beautiful women. But I'd never fallen in love. Before he died, Big Pun used to joke that he fell in love with every woman he ever met—which always made me laugh because, as much as I liked girls, I had never had it happen to me. There were always girls around the way in Hollis who liked me, but that was usually the extent of my dealings with women. The moment I saw Zuri, though, life instantly became about something much more.

I was twenty-seven at the time. She wasn't even quite eighteen yet. I remember how she walked, how she moved, her mannerisms. She was just way more mature than the other girls she was with, and some of them were in their early twenties. I stepped to her, asked her what her name was, and struck up a brief conversation. She knew who I was, but because she was ten years younger, the whole Run-DMC thing didn't really mean that much to her. New Edition, LL Cool J, and everything that had come after us was what she was really into. She'd grown up in Hartford, Connecticut, so all she really knew was KISS-FM, pop music, soul, R&B. She liked hip-hop, but she definitely wasn't tripping because I was an MC. I liked that. We chatted for a minute. I got her phone number and promised her that I was going to call. I found out later that when I walked away, her friends had to convince her that I was actually flirting with her. They were like, "DMC's hitting on you! When that man calls you, you'd better pick up the phone!" Then she went home and told her sister, Jackie, who's my age, that "I met the DMC guy." Her sister flipped out, but Zuri still wasn't a fan.

I called her the next day, and we talked for a while. I visited her the day after that because I was flying to Europe the following day. It was like I just *had* to see this woman before I left. I went by, we talked, laughed. I realized that whatever sensation had put thoughts of marriage in my head wasn't something that was going to pass. I was in love with her at first sight. The next day, I went to Europe for two weeks. When I came back home, she was the first person I called. We went out either the day I got back or the next day, and we've been at each other's side and have had each other's back ever since.

Dating her was great. She opened me up to a new world. Back then, she was a background dancer on *Club MTV*, a show that was hosted by Downtown Julie Brown. She was also trying to sing in some girl group that wanted to be the next En Vogue. She had dropped out of school and was attending night school to get her diploma while she was dancing on MTV during the day and singing. At the time, I was sober and not going to clubs anymore, so I just fell into her world. I would take her up to MTV so she could do her TV stuff. Meanwhile, I was there sitting around talking to all these executives I'd made history with when "Rock Box" broke down the barriers that had kept rap off TV. Her friends would be tripping—"Oh my God, that's DMC." Later, I would take her over to Jersey for her night classes.

We did normal stuff like driving around the city, something I'd always liked to do. Although I wasn't drinking anymore, sometimes I would get a bag of chronic, and I'd let Zuri drive us around for hours while I smoked. She was wise beyond her years even then, so it was always easy for me to just sit up, smoke, and have these long conversations with her. Other times, I took her to the salon to get her nails done. Or I would take her and her mother shopping. As unbelievable as it might seem, a lot of this was new to me! Remember, Run-DMC blew up when we were like nineteen, twenty years old. I came straight out of high school and into showbiz. My life hadn't been like the average twenty-one-, twenty-two-, twenty-three-year-old dude who might spend time with his girl. I had missed out on some of the mundane things that guys my age do with their girlfriends, so I was catching up. It was a completely different scene, and I enjoyed it all.

I began making little changes based on what she liked. I remember she once told me that I was getting too skinny, so I cut back on dieting and started lifting more weights. Maybe the biggest change, though, was when she asked me one day to take off my glasses. I remember her studying my face for a long time, and then saying, "I love you with your glasses, but I think you look good without them." My glasses, of course, had been a big part of my identity as DMC. (Most people thought I wore Cazals, which were *the* popular brand when we first started out. In truth, though, I never wore Cazals; I wore a brand called Ultra Goliath.) Ever since our first album, on songs like "Hollis Crew (Krush Groove 2)," we had spit verses like, *"And why you wear those glasses? / So I can see."* We had songs like "You're Blind," in which we said shit like, *"You're blind / You can't see / You need to wear some glasses like DMC."* But when she told me that, I started to not wear them as much. But, of course, I'm blind as a bat, so I had to go get contacts. As much as my glasses had meant to my image, I had no reservations about giving them up. It was time. I wasn't drinking anymore. I had cut off all my hair. I had entered into a new reality. With her, I was discovering a life I never knew existed. I was going through some real transformative superhero shit. It was like when Peter Parker switched from the red-and-blue Spider-Man suit to the all-black joint!

Anytime I wasn't in the studio or on the road, I was with Zuri. As soon as I'd get back home, she was the first person I'd call. She never got upset about my schedule or my traveling. She understood. Plus, she was young, so she had her own life. In many ways, her life was busier than mine. I only had about four things to do—hit the studio, do a radio interview, perform a show, and go home. She had a million other things to keep her busy. Plus, she really didn't care about all that shit anyway. When we would perform nearby, she didn't come to the shows back then. She really, honestly, was not a fan. It was lucky for both of us.

We dated for about a year, and then, in 1993, we got married. Our ceremony was a small, private one, held at the civil courthouse on Queens Boulevard near my old neighborhood in Hollis. It was me, my wife, her best friend, and her mom. We jumped the broom! Not long after we were hitched, I moved us to a house in New Jersey, since that's where my wife had been living with her mom ever since her mom had divorced her dad and had come down from Connecticut. Our son, who we named D'Son (after all, he was "D.'s son"), was born the next year.

I haven't always had a great sense of what it means to be a dad. I've always traveled a lot, so I've spent far more time away from my son than I'd like. In fact, I used to travel so much that when his teachers in school would ask him what his daddy did for a living, he'd tell them I was a pilot! It was kind of cute, but kind of sad, too. All he ever knew was that Daddy was always getting dropped off at and picked up from the airport, so he just assumed I flew the planes.

But as my son has gotten older, we've gotten closer. He spends more time out on the road with me now. He's getting a chance to see who I am away from the house. He was born after I stopped drinking the first time, and he was a little guy when I relapsed, so he doesn't know much about me when I was at my worst. And that's a good thing. I wouldn't have wanted him to see me like that.

Now he gets to see me as the self-assured, centered person who's emerged from all my troubles. He doesn't know much about the emotional wreck I used to be, but he sees how I refuse to be bogged down by drama and other people's baggage. He jokes about it like, "Daddy will ignore everybody!" I don't ignore people, but I also don't let other people's problems poison my well-being anymore. I'm actually glad to be able to model that attitude for my son.

When it came to my career, Zuri was always very supportive, even though she wasn't into our music. My family adored her. My crew loved her, too, which made things that much easier. There was no skepticism, never any fear that she was trying to home in on my fame or take advantage of my money. People knew from the very beginning of our relationship that she was sincere in her love for me. They also knew that I felt likewise, and almost everyone made an effort to embrace her. She got along great with Jay. Zuri and Jay's girlfriend, Terri, clicked right away and became very close. It wasn't hard to like her.

One thing she would say to me, though, was that she wanted to punch that motherfucker Run in his face. She saw Run as very disrespectful toward people. To her, he was arrogant and bossy and acted like he was better. She thought he wanted, more than anything else, to control people—especially me. So they didn't always get along but were usually cordial.

Zuri came into my life as it was undergoing profound changes. Run needed me for the tours and the spot dates and the interviews. He saw that things were changing when my wife came along. I wasn't caring as much about being a team player or about helping him with his agenda. Before that, I didn't have any kids or steady girlfriends, and was at his beck and call. He could go home to his family and be gone from the group as long as he wanted and never expected us to say anything about it. But now that I had something else that was taking up my time, it was driving him crazy.

It used to be, when we came off the road, like during

the *Raising Hell* and *Tougher than Leather* tours, we'd have three or four days to do normal stuff, or maybe an interview. I never saw him any other time, but he would call me at eight thirty in the morning, saying, "D., I'm on my way to pick you up right now. We got to go to Russell's." "We got to go to see Mr. Magic." "We got to go to see Funkmaster Flex." "We got to go to Profile."

But now it was, "D., we got to—"

And I'd be cutting him off: "I can't do it today, man." It's urgent for Run, of course, because he's got to get back to his wife and kids and his life. So it's, "We need to do this now" because he's only got this window from, say, eleven a.m. to one thirty or whatever. So it's, "I need to use you to get this accomplished." But I was not available. I had other obligations. He was losing control, and he hated it. I can imagine that's probably why he went bald. He was probably pulling his hair out because shit got different. It became apparent real fast that I had other priorities.

Zuri was the first time I'd had something in my life that was more important than music or being in Run-DMC. Loving Zuri also forced me over the years to love myself better. My evolution took years, even after I met her, but she was a big part of what inspired me to want to be better, to want to overcome the health struggles and addiction and rage and depression that had straitjacketed my life.

I've learned self-love through my love for Zuri. As a

result, I've learned my true value. I've learned that my value isn't in how many records I've sold or how many concert arenas I've filled or how many awards I've won. We can't define ourselves simply by how much money we've made or how well we've done on the job or in school. I realize now that my value is in my ideas, my willingness to share in order to help others, my ever-growing desire to stand firm on an issue and not back down. Knowing your value is part of defining yourself. When you don't realize that value, you allow other people to make you into what *they* want you to be—even if that thing isn't healthy for you.

As a member of Run-DMC, I had so many ideas that I wanted to bring to the table, so many ways that I wanted to contribute. But I let other people—I'm not going to blame others for what I allowed—tell me what was significant about what I had to offer. I let other people tell me that I just had to be DMC the B-boy or DMC the hard rhymer. I never gave myself a chance to break out of other people's molds until I'd nearly destroyed my body, my future, and my mind. When you lowball your value, you also deny other people the chance to benefit from what you have to bring. What if I'd been able to do more with our group during the *Tougher Than Leather* and *Back from Hell* and *Crown Royal* projects? Sure, I might've failed, too. Our career might've still gone down a hole—but at least I'd have had a hand in taking it down that hole. I wasn't drinking because we were failing. I was drinking because I wasn't a full participant in that failure, if you can understand that. Even when you lose, you want to feel like you count.

But then again, had I been allowed to do more, we might've had more success. There might not have been a *Back from Hell*. We might not have had to wait for Pete Rock to save us or for Jason Nevins to make us hot again. Me dressing up, doing the Running Man in videos, all that shit was uncalled for. *Back from Hell* was destined to fail because Jay was writing all the music, and Run was giving all the directions. Who knows how I might've affected our destiny if I'd recognized a larger sense of purpose? The worst part is, we'll never know—because I never forced anyone to respect the full breadth of what I had to offer. The DMC part of me had so much more to give, but because I wasn't forcing anyone to recognize and utilize that treasure, that gem, that existence, became worthless to me.

You can't love yourself properly when you're feeding yourself negativity. You can't buy into other people's poor perceptions of you. You can't get caught up in trying to please someone else by repressing your own goals or wants or feelings.

Loving yourself means realizing you're greater than the title on your business card or the grades on a school progress report. Whatever you think your purpose is in life now, know that it isn't necessarily your destiny, and destiny isn't purpose. It's not like we were put here to do just one thing in life or stay somewhere once we've arrived. Destiny can be many points on a spectrum, not just one. I wasn't put here to be the "King of Rock." That was just something I achieved along the way. Eminem once said that nobody in hip-hop will ever do what me, Run, and Jay did. That's very cool to say, but my destiny isn't determined by those achievements. My destiny could change any day once I start applying my skill or talent to be used for a specific purpose.

I was doing some audio drops for an African American history segment and had the opportunity to tell someone who I was working with that I'd recently felt free to speak my truth. Consequently, I no longer had to worry about what was going to happen to me day to day. I could speak freely, be me, and enjoy just that. It's almost like when I was writing rhymes in my mother's basement in Hollis as a kid. I didn't know what was going to happen, and I didn't really care. I was doing what I enjoyed. I didn't necessarily have a purpose for doing it, but I was able to discover one purpose for which I had been created. I found purpose more than purpose found me.

I lost my voice—but in the years since, I've found that I have reached and touched even more people, in a much realer way, than ever before. I lost my voice but have never been heard with the force and volume with which I'm able to speak today. Run-DMC was my destiny. Now working with adoptees, orphans, and foster kids is my destiny. Destiny doesn't have permanency. Purpose just keeps destiny coming at you, keeps you moving through all those different points on that spectrum. Purpose can keep you alive, no matter what you may think your destiny is. And love gives one the greatest purpose of all.

When we're hurt or angry, our mind and body are trying to get us to respond to whatever external factors are producing those feelings. But if we're drowning out those messages with alcohol or drugs, all we're really doing is furthering our inability to deal with a problem. People who abuse drugs often do so to cope with something. But coping with an issue isn't the same thing as addressing an issue, and it's certainly not the same as fixing an issue. You need clarity to fix the problems you face. Having that clarity means, above everything else, being real, not just with others, but with yourself. That is a huge part of self-love.

Finding Zuri expanded my ability to love. After I met her, it grew deeper. My self-love grew through my love of her. By that I mean I learned that I had to take better care of myself to fully love her the way that she deserves. Learning to give the highest level of love that you have to somebody is a gift to yourself and to the person who you are sharing it with.

Of course, it's never easy when you're trying to love someone who's been in the midst of intense personal evolution for years, as I have. I'm not exactly the same guy my wife married back in '93. When she met me, our group was trying to salvage our career. Since we've been together, I've joined and left the church, found out I was adopted, relapsed into drinking, gone through deep depression, thought about killing myself, checked into rehab, undergone intensive therapy, and embraced a whole new way of being and seeing the world. I'm more honest than I've ever been, which is a trip for her, because she wasn't always used to me saying what was on my mind.

If I'm being honest, I can't say my healing and changing have always been great for my marriage. It's like as soon as my wife gets acclimated to me being one way, something crazy happens. (Like when she goes on the road, she doesn't think it's very fun. I tell her, "It was fun *before* you got here.") But since she's been in my life, it's taken some drastic changes. I went from church to this alcohol shit. Now from the alcohol shit it goes to this new dude who is determined to make decisions. She's learning to understand that I'm fluid. I can be stubborn, but if something doesn't work out one way, I'll switch up.

But what doesn't change is that I love her deeply.

Love is the most powerful emotion there is. When it is real, it transforms your life for the better. It makes you smile. It makes you feel good. It makes you put your best foot forward. This is what I have experienced in having a loving wife and son. They have become my everything. They give me the strength to deal with my depression and to keep it in check, which is important.

At my worst, I used to think they would be fine without me, that my unresolved emotional troubles were only ruining their lives. But I think that, even though I didn't openly acknowledge it then, having them was a big reason why I didn't put a gun to my head and pull the trigger. My loving relationship with Zuri and D'Son have shown me that the purpose for all human beings is to love each other, to give love, and through that love heal each other of emotional pain. Love is the best soothing balm.

TEN

REMIXED

BRINGING OUT THE
BEST IN ME

'**ve got issues. So do you.**

Money or a lack of it doesn't change the fact that we all have issues. Neither does fame. I don't care who you are, where you've gone, or what you've seen. No amount of life experience or money or privilege is going to lighten the load of the baggage that we lug around.

No matter how damaged I felt, I had an obligation to myself and my family to address the internal flaws that threatened my life. I could not afford to tolerate them or try to hold them at bay. Coping with my issues in life wasn't the same as fixing them. I learned the hard way that just because I could stop drinking, it did not mean I could cope with the problems that were at the root of my drinking. Sitting quietly in a room when I felt disrespected or unfairly ignored wasn't any better than guzzling forty ounces of crappy beer when it came to addressing these feelings.

Most of us need someone to talk with as a form of seeking help. We need counseling, therapy. It is not a sign of weakness to seek help. Life is complex and subtle and insidious, in that problems often accumulate quietly, festering inside you for years sometimes before you realize how serious they've become. At the same time, to complicate matters more, changes are taking place within us all the time. If we're not diligently scrutinizing, critiquing, and bettering ourselves, incremental damages can sneak up on us. But work hard enough, desire a goal enough, put enough pressure on yourself, and you can at least start the process of working through whatever troubles you.

I'm still trying to repair myself. I always will be, in a lot of respects. I work on myself in all aspects of my life, because being whole means just that—fixing all of you. Therapy has taught me that anger and resentment are like acid. Holding on to them just corrodes me from the inside. I can remember the long years of silently simmering at the world. Even when I was sober, I kept so many negative feelings pent up inside me that I felt weighed down every day. They weren't just negative feelings about others. The worst of these feelings I often directed at myself. I allowed myself to be victimized by circumstances that I should've taken control of, but didn't, and I became consumed with bitterness and regret.

After I shattered under the weight of my problems, I began the long process of piecing myself back together. Exercise helped. My counseling sessions with professionals like Wendy Freund were critical. But I also found relief in other, sometimes surprising, ways.

One example is how I ran across "Angel," the song that, as I explained earlier, helped save my life. I had arrived home from a trip in 1996. I came out of JFK airport, got in the car, and the young-dude driver said, "Oh, shit!" He was impressed that DMC was his passenger. The whole time he was driving, he kept peeking at me in the rearview mirror. When I'd look up at him, he'd turn his head like he was looking elsewhere. Eventually, we stopped at a red light and he fully turned around to look at me. "I'm not supposed to do this. I might get fired, but, yo, I got to take a picture. I love Run-DMC." I never, ever have a problem with taking pictures with fans. I've always been grateful to anybody who listens to our music and appreciates what we do. "Sure, whatever you want." We took a picture before continuing on our journey. I was quiet, caught up in my own world of problems, when the driver asked if it would be OK if he turned on the radio. (In fancy cars they ask. In ghetto cars it's on blast before you even get in, and you have to yell for the driver to hear your requested destination!) I said, "Yeah, whatever." He turned it to Hot 97, the hip-hop station. The last thing I wanted to hear was hip-hop. Since I couldn't rhyme anymore, I didn't even want to hear it.

The station had Busta Rhymes or Method Man or someone like that on. There was a bunch of people being interviewed on Funkmaster Flex's show, and all of these dudes were talking about the commercialization of hip-hop. I couldn't take it.

"Don't turn it there, please," I said. "Can you try something else? *Anything* else."

He looked at me kinda funny at first—*how the fuck does a rap legend not want to listen to the hip-hop station?*—but then he obliged and turned it to this Lite FM station, WPLJ. The station often took me back to some of my earliest exposure to music on the radio, when I was a kid listening to Credence Clearwater Revival and Harry Chapin. Now, though, it wasn't those songs that touched me. The song that was playing on the radio was one that I'd never heard before, one that went right to my soul as soon as I heard it. It moved me in ways I had never been moved before. Oddly, as I wallowed in my own pain and sorrow and self-pity, it was just the song I needed to hear.

"Angel" is a piano record—dark and heavy. Right then and there, cruising through the bustling city, just home from Europe, I felt that song speak to me like no other. It felt like Sarah McLachlan had recorded that song specifically for me and I was meant to hear it at that very moment.

I woke up the next morning with my wife at my side. "Hey, honey, you heard of Sarah McLachlan, that song 'Angel'? I really like it." I mentioned it to her because anything I say that I like, my wife likes to get it and surprise me. Sure enough, the next day I had the whole Sarah McLachlan album. Over the next year, that was the song I listened to every day, "Angel," all day, on repeat. I listened to all the other songs on the album, "Building a Mystery," this and that. Then I went out and bought everything she'd ever recorded.

For a whole year, every day I listened to "Angel" for almost the entire day. Wherever I was and whatever I was doing, the song was with me. Sometimes, I didn't even want to leave my house for listening to that song. When the guys would come and pick me up for a gig, I had the song in my possession and they had to listen to it, too. When I got into the car I would tell my crew, "Yo, you got to play this," and hand them "Angel." After a while, Smith and Jay began protesting: "We ain't playing that song!"

When they would refuse to play the song, I would turn around and walk back into the house.

Erik, my manager, made them realize that I wasn't joking around. "That motherfucker's serious, yo!" "All right, D. All right." I'd sit in the limo, humming the song. They got sick of it, but I didn't care. I *needed* that record.

It would be too simple to say that song got rid of all my negative feelings and pain and resentment, because that's not what happened. It couldn't rid me of the wounds or of that strange, inexplicable, gnawing void that was compounding all the hurt and rejection I'd endured. "Angel" was like a life preserver tossed to me in an ocean during a storm. It didn't pull me out of the water, but it did help me stay afloat until other help came along.

I fell in love with "Angel" during my deep depression in the late 1990s, and several months after I first heard it I got a chance to actually meet the woman whose song had had such an impact on me. We met at a Grammy party thrown by the record executive Clive Davis in 1997.

Erik called me one day to tell me that he'd landed tickets to Clive's bash, which was a very big deal in the music industry. He was excited about it, too, as tickets to Clive's parties weren't easy to come by, even for star recording artists. As excited as he was, though, I was equally as uninterested. I couldn't have cared less about anything related to the music business at that point, especially not parties. The fame, the glamor, the money, to my mind, were all nonsense. Erik, who is usually a very laid-back guy, was audibly annoyed by my lack of concern. He and Tracey Miller, Run-DMC's publicist, had pulled some pretty big strings to get those tickets. "Yo, D., you need to go," he said. "It'll be real big. Tracey Miller set this up."

"I don't care," I told him. "I ain't going."

"D., I worked real hard to get these tickets."

Erik had to resort to explaining that he'd promised Tracey that I'd show up. I still acted like I didn't care anything about it. Erik repeated his plea. "D., you don't know how hard I worked to get these tickets. I told Tracey you were going."

"You shouldn't have told her that," I replied coolly.

Erik has always stood by me, through some of the best and worst times in my life. Even before he became our manager, he used to tote around coolers filled with my 40-ounces. It wasn't a high-profile job by any means, but he did it with the same seriousness and commitment that he does almost everything. Erik had paid dues and has remained a loyal friend, even when I've given him a hard time. For that, he has always merited my respect. Furthermore, he's as business-savvy a dude as he is a devoted friend, which makes me listen to him when he talks, even if it takes me some time to come around. I knew that he was angry at me because of the way I was acting, but in spite of his being upset, he stayed after me about that party until the date finally arrived a couple of weeks later.

"OK, I'll go," I said. "But I'm only staying for one hour."

"That's fine with me," he said. "All you have to do is walk the red carpet and take a couple of pictures."

"I ain't doing all of that, but I will go to the party."

On our way to the opulent Beverly Hills Hotel, where the party was being thrown, I swore to him that I wasn't staying longer than an hour. I meant it, too. I was supposed to sit at some VIP table, but I took a table near a back corner of the room instead. It was as close to the exit as I could get. As soon as I sat down, I glanced at my watch and began the minute-by-minute countdown to the moment when I could bounce. *Fifty-nine . . . fifty-eight . . . fifty-seven . . .* If I could've speeded up time, I would have gladly done so.

As the party picked up, the major stars who always attend Clive's gigs filed in—Stevie Wonder, Alicia Keys, Busta Rhymes, P. Diddy, and the like. I stared around with an almost glazed look in my eyes. I was as unmoved as I'd been when Erik first invited me. Meanwhile, people were walking up to my table showing me nothing but love, telling me how young I looked and asking for the secret to my youth. I made nice, but in the back of my mind, all I could think about was going back to my hotel room, cranking up "Angel," and reading books on metaphysics or something.

On my behalf, Erik was working the room, selecting particular media personalities who he wanted to have interview me on the red carpet. Usually, I was happy to talk to an entire pressroom full of reporters. This night, though, I probably spoke to maybe only three journalists total. That had to be some kind of all-time low for me. Then, minutes after I wrapped up my last interview and was about to resume my countdown, I looked up, and what I saw nearly made my eyes pop out of their sockets.

Sarah McLachlan had walked in.

Since I was near the door, I was the first person to see her as she strolled into the room. "Oh my God, that's her,"

I said, gasping. I couldn't stop staring as she walked across the room, speaking with small groups of people.

I wanted to rush over to her, but I hesitated. Only a few people knew I was a closet Sarah McLachlan fan—and almost none of them were at this party. I thought briefly of how it might look to others to see the "King of Rock" fawning over a pop soloist. I quickly said, "Forget that." This woman had helped save my life. As I saw that she was about to head into a larger room that was swarming with industry bigwigs, I feared that I might never get another chance to tell her what her music meant to me. Nervous and excited, I quickly made my way over to where she was standing. When I opened my mouth to speak, I sounded nothing like the swaggering rap superhero I projected on-stage and in videos. My tone softened considerably.

"Excuse me, Ms. McLachlan," I started meekly.

She turned around, saw it was me, and allowed a giant grin to spread across her face. "DMC? Oh, Run-DMC, I love you guys!"

Surprisingly, she began to actually rhyme the lyrics to some of our songs. It was a medley of Run-DMC classics. *"It's tricky to rock a rhyme/to rock a rhyme that's right on time."* *"My Ahhh-didas walk through concert doors/and roam all over coliseum floors."* She sounded damn good, too. I was beyond flattered. I even thought, *OK, that's a good reason to stay alive. Sarah McLachlan likes my group's music.*

Jittery with nerves, my tongue drying out with

each word, I continued: "That's so cool, thank you. Well, Ms. McLachlan, I just want to tell you that one of your records saved my life. This past year I've been depressed and suicidal. I listen to that record every day. It's the crutch that I stand on. I don't leave my house without listening to that record. I don't work out without listening to that record. I don't travel without listening to that record. The name of the record is 'Angel,' and you sing like an angel. People say you are an angel, but you're not an angel to me. You're a god."

I must've babbled on like that for more than two minutes. When I finished, I could see bafflement all over her face. Clearly, she hadn't expected me to pour out my heart all over the floor in front of her at the hottest party of the year. I'm sure the poor woman simply intended to say hello, pay me a compliment, and keep it moving. She was gracious about it, nonetheless. She shook my hand, looked me in my eyes, and said, "Thank you for telling me that, Darryl—but that's what music is supposed to do."

I was overjoyed.

I will never forget that meeting.

GRADUALLY, OVER THE next two years, I tried to make my way to a place where I could handle my issues maturely and effectively. I was tired of the emotional roller coaster that I was on and wanted permanent healing. The first action I took was owning my talent. After years of stagnation, I was feeling creative again. I was becoming more serious about putting out a solo album, which took me in and out of various studios over the following few years. I sifted through tracks, laid a plethora of vocals, and plotted everything from my new stage show to how I'd market myself. I even signed a deal with a small label, Roman Empire Records.

While working on my music, I was influenced by many people and various events in my life. No matter what I was going through, there were always good people in my life. When I wanted to get well, the good people proved instrumental in helping lift me up. One big influence was—and has continued to be—my friend Sheila Jaffe, who I've known since 2000. I was introduced to her by an entertainment agent. He and I were having a conversation about a work project, and it quickly turned into me venting about being adopted and not having anyone I could share my new feelings with. As the agent and I talked—really, I did all the talking and he just listened with interest—he suddenly began scrolling through the contacts in his cell phone.

Once I stopped complaining, he looked over at me and told me there was someone he wanted me to meet. "Last week Sheila Jaffe was in here, and it sounds like you two have so much in common—you two have to meet!"

I met Sheila for dinner and almost immediately we began talking about how we could use our experiences to help other adoptees. Then, as we were wrapping up, she told me, "Darryl, if you ever need to come to any discussion groups, once a month, fellow adoptees and I get together—it's nothing big but we just sit and talk about adoption." I couldn't wait to go, because until then, it seemed to me that I was the only person in the world struggling with being adopted.

At the first support-group meeting, I realized I was far from alone. Suddenly I was part of a community. I returned every month to hear more.

Sheila and I also helped start a support group for young people called the Felix Organization. As part of our work, we send about two hundred kids a year from New York City to a five-week summer camp. There's swimming, rock climbing, nature, basketball, arts and crafts, dance, yoga, and DJs. We expose the kids to a multitude of artistic, creative, and educational careers. We got so good that, in our second year, the New York School of Dance heard what we were doing and said, "We're going to come up there and teach the kids for free." It's worked out so well that our camp even produced one girl who was so superbly gifted the dance school agreed to send her to school for free.

Let me tell you, that work hasn't been easy—but it's been more fulfilling to me than anything else I've done. We've reached more than two thousand kids over the past ten years, and that's more meaningful than any hit record or music award I've ever enjoyed. We haven't saved them all. I had one kid recently who had been in the program for years, and had even become a counselor after he aged out of the program. I found out not long ago that he killed himself. Broke my heart, man. But it also made me that much more determined to help save as many others as I can. Starting that group, working on behalf of adoptees, that was an integral part of my recovery.

Even as I was growing into an advocate for adoptees, though, I was also still trying to figure out how to best use my music to heal. On my solo album, I was determined to make songs that would help orphans, foster kids, and adopted kids who were grasping for identity and purpose, same as I was. I wanted to make a song that would affirm, uplift, and encourage them the same way Sarah McLachlan's music had done for me. I wanted to be someone's "angel," too.

I thought about the kind of music that would help underscore an affirming message. I thought back to songs I enjoyed when I was a child. As much as I'd loved the soul and R&B records that my friends, family, and neighbors always played, I also had an unusual attraction to rock 'n' roll, especially thoughtful, introspective music. Sure, I dug the Jackson Five, Sly and the Family Stone, and James Brown as a kid, just like most of the other kids on my block, but I also listened to the Beatles, Bob Dylan, John Lennon, and Elton John. As a child, some of my favorite songs had been pop records like "Bad, Bad Leroy Brown" by Jim Croche,

"Yellow Submarine" by the Beatles, and "Cat's in the Cradle" by Harry Chapin. As I rifled through my mental playlist, the Chapin song kept coming back to me. I thought about how melancholy that song is, how it told the story of a father who never had time to spend with his son.

I decided I would tell my own story—about a little boy who was given up for adoption and how two loving parents adopted him and gave him life—to that Harry Chapin song. Then, out of nowhere, another idea struck me. It came so hard, so fast, that I actually blurted it out loud to myself. "I'm going to ask Sarah McLachlan to do that record with me!" If I was going to try to be an "angel" to someone else, it only made sense that I collaborate with the songstress who'd been that for me.

Right after the idea hit me, I called up Erik: "I need to get in touch with Sarah McLachlan because I'm going to do a remake of 'Cat's in the Cradle,' and I want her on the song with me. See if you can find out how to contact her so I can ask."

Erik ain't know who in the world Harry Chapin even was. I'm sure he thought, *Whatever makes crazy-ass D. happy.* As always, he didn't ask many questions. He just went to work. A few days later, as usual, Erik came through for me. I was at dinner with my wife at one of our favorite restaurants when my cell phone rang: "Yo, D., you have to call Sarah McLachlan right now. She's waiting for you."

I took down Sarah's number and walked outside to

make the call in private. I was real nervous, worrying that she might turn me down, especially after I dumped my feelings all over her at that Grammy party in 1997. I dialed the number and she answered the phone. "Hey, Ms. McLachlan, this is Darryl, do you remember me?"

"How can I forget you? You called me God," she said. "What's up?"

Now I'm thinking, *If she thought I was crazy back then, she's really going to think I'm crazy now.* "Remember when I met you three years ago and I told you what your record did for me?" I asked.

"Yeah, I remember that."

"And then you told me that's what music was supposed to do."

"Yeah."

"Well, I found out why I was going through all the stuff that I was going through. I had just found out that I was adopted. My mother brought me home when I was one month old, and I want to make a record that will help people the way that your record helped me. . . . And I would like to know if you'd agree to do the record with me."

Her answer came quick, without even a half second of hesitation: "Yes, I will."

I was so excited that I screamed into the other phone where Erik was still waiting for me: "Yo, Erik, she said she'll do it!"

"D., talk to *her*! You're going to lose her," replied Erik.

I hadn't figured out what I'd say to her after I asked her to record with me. To me, it was such a long shot that I was expecting her to turn me down flat. I hastily put together a plan. "Ms. McLachlan, we'll fly you to New York City, put you up in the Four Seasons Hotel—"

She interrupted. "No, no, no, Darryl. You don't have to do all of that. You can come to my house in Vancouver to make the record. I have a studio in my house."

I was stunned. I thought I was going to pass out or some shit. I started making plans to get to Vancouver immediately.

Several days later, on the plane to Vancouver, I turned to Erik and said, "If I die tomorrow . . ."

Erik couldn't stand to hear me talk like that. After seeing me go through my suicidal period and after enduring the death of Jay, he always feared that I was secretly wishing death on myself. He cut me short and said, "Don't say that."

I pressed on, yelling at him now: "NOW YOU LISTEN TO ME!" Stunned, he just stared back at me and nodded.

"If I die tomorrow," I resumed, "you let the world know it wasn't the gold or platinum records. It wasn't being on MTV. It wasn't being DMC. The best thing to happen to me in my music career is making a record with Sarah McLachlan."

I meant it, too. Her record had had deep significance for me, and I felt like the record she and I were about to make together would one day have deep meaning to someone else. I didn't care *how many* people it touched. I wasn't looking for the song to go gold or platinum. If only one person got something out of it, that would be the greatest success I could hope for. *Run-DMC*, *King of Rock*, and *Raising Hell* had affected millions of listeners, so I knew what it was like to have commercial triumph and global adulation. I didn't need that anymore, and I certainly didn't need it with our record. I wanted this record to save a life, to uplift someone's spirit, to explain to an orphaned girl wondering about her birth parents or a little boy in foster care that I knew how they felt and that, despite their circumstances, they still mattered and still had a purpose. I decided to call the song "Just Like Me."

I spent two days in Vancouver cutting "Just Like Me" with Sarah. She brought in her band, introduced me to her family, and treated me and Erik like we were her long-lost friends. When the song was done and we were ready to leave to catch our flight home, she walked us to the door and told me to give her team a couple of days to mix the record. Of course, that wasn't an issue, as I was simply grateful to have had the chance to work with her, and I said as much. As we entered the foyer of her house, she stopped walking, and stopped talking. She took a seat. She drew in a deep breath, gazed up at me, and said, "But before you go, Darryl, I want to tell you something. You probably didn't know this, but I was adopted, too."

Truthfully, I don't know what the fuck I said in response to that, don't know how I reacted. I was numb and dazed. I just remember saying good-bye and walking out of Sarah McLachlan's house slowly, like some kind of zombie. Later, as Erik, the record label executives, and I began to digest what she'd just revealed, we got a collective case of the chills. She could've told me that information over the phone, but she clearly was still dealing with whatever her own adoption situation had been.

After I got back to New York, she and I talked about doing a video to accompany the record. As we worked out the details, her manager, Terry McBride, told me something that gave me even more faith that our record could help someone.

"People ask Sarah to do stuff all the time, but that was the quickest I've ever heard Sarah go with a yes," he said. "She said she'll do the video, and she'll do press with you, whatever you need to do. But she doesn't want to take questions about her adoption situation."

I completely understood. I could only hope that working on this record had helped her in some way, too. I think that's why she asked me out to her home in Vancouver. She knew this record was special. She knew it had the potential to bring light to the lives of orphans and adoptees and foster kids whose own lives had been marked by turmoil as they struggled to find themselves.

THE EXPERIENCES WITH Sarah and Sheila Jaffe were enlightening. Deep down, though, it was still a fight for me to care about my life. When I first got married, I wasn't drinking. But, in later years, I went back to the bottle. My wife said I was drinking in excess to cover up my sadness and confusion over being adopted.

I recall attending the Billboard Music Awards one year during my relapse and being at a bar. This middle-aged white dude walked up to me, saw me tossing back shots, and immediately registered concern. He'd checked out my first book, *King of Rock: Respect, Responsibility, and My Life with Run-DMC*, which by the end gives the reader the impression that all was well with me. Clearly, it wasn't, and this guy could tell. "Are you supposed to be drinking?" His words caught me by surprise, and they cut deep. My alcohol buzz evaporated on the spot, and I remember getting really upset. Fortunately for us both, I have never been a violent drunk, because I might've actually punched him. Instead, I stalked off, knowing full well that I was mad at him only because he had spoken the truth. Not ready to face the truth, I moved on to another bar where I could drink in peace.

I recall being in Japan in early 2004 for a promotional

trip. My solo album, which I'd titled *Checks Thugs and Rock N Roll*, was nearly ready, and I had gone overseas to meet with the head of Sony and to do some press. While there, I met a woman who worked for MTV Japan. She owned this cool scooter that she rode around town. I asked her if I could take it for a test spin—even though I was drunk as shit. At first, she was hesitant. Erik was with me and silently motioned to the woman to not let me drive. I kept pressing her and she relented.

I crashed it almost immediately. The woman was in tears, as I had completely wrecked her means of transportation. I covered the damages, of course. But, in that moment, standing face-to-face with the crying woman, I realized that I needed serious help.

The very next day, I met with members of the Japanese music press. I was still hungover from the night before, but I was managing to get through the interviews OK. Most of the questions were noninvasive and friendly and complimentary of my music and my history as a hip-hop groundbreaker. But then, in what was probably the next-to-last interview of the day, a reporter who'd heard some tracks from the solo album stuck a mic in my face and asked me outright, "DMC, are you OK?" I told her I was. I thought she might've noticed my hungover look or, worse, found out about the drunken scooter episode from the day before. She said, "This solo album you've done, it's very dark."

Nobody else had asked anything remotely close to

that, and it forced me to pause. I realized that I didn't really even know what was on the album. I had been so drunk and so hurt throughout so much of the process that I had been recording lyrics that I couldn't even totally remember. In fact, there was one song that I'd done with DJ Lethal that I couldn't remember writing or rhyming. I was so blinded to my own pain that it took someone else to see my darkness.

When the last interviewer stepped up, he asked me if there was anything I wished I'd done differently on my solo debut.

"Yeah," I told him, the previous reporter's comments still working their way through my head. "I wish I'd have made a happier record."

I wasn't sure how successful I'd be at making new music or starting on the comic book project I had dreamed of for so long. Once I got a handle on the revelation that I was adopted, I tried to use that to my advantage, too, resolving to share my stories with others who had grown up in orphanages and foster homes and with adoptive families. I began traveling the country to make speeches to orphaned children nationwide, and I remain a committed adoption advocate to this day. I've found greater purpose than I ever imagined back when I was shut up in hotel rooms thinking my life had reached its end.

I live freely these days, no longer saddled with other people's expectations or definitions of me. I live honestly. I don't keep quiet when I should speak, or lie when I know

I need to articulate my truth. I don't drink or use drugs at all. I don't need crutches. I don't retreat into a shell to hide in anymore. I stand on my own, honestly and in full view of the world. I'm not alone, and I refuse to live like that for even one more day.

Making the album was therapy for me. I worked out a lot of anger and a lot of deep-seated pain. It was cathartic to be able to lash out musically, even if some of my anger was misdirected. Recording that album during those dark years in 2002 and 2003 was my release, my sounding board, my punching bag. You know how when an athlete gets hurt and someone documents the rehab? When I look back on making *Checks Thugs and Rock N Roll*, I see that it was part of my rehab. The beautiful thing about *Checks Thugs and Rock N Roll* was that it allowed me to get back on the horse by keeping me working, which kept me sane. When the album was released in the United States in 2006, the critics trashed it.

BY EARLY 2003, everyone around me who cared, from my friends to my wife to my manager, was urging me to go get help. It wasn't until after I went to Las Vegas for a New Year's Eve show that I decided to take their advice. After I finished performing that night with my man DJ Hurricane, I went back to my hotel room alone. There, sitting by myself, I drank an entire fifth of Rémy Martin cognac.

When I sobered up the next day, I looked at that big, empty bottle and made up my mind right then and there that I was going to change. If I didn't, I knew I wasn't going to last much longer. Finally I cared about living, which was an accomplishment in and of itself. "I'm going to rehab," I told myself.

Surprisingly, as soon as I started making real plans to go to rehab, I stopped drinking immediately. I was scheduled to check myself into the rehabilitation clinic in April, and for the entire month of March I didn't drink. The norm is for someone to go on a bender or use their hardest just before they enter rehab, sort of as a last hurrah before giving themselves over to sobriety. I was the opposite. I wanted to go into rehab ready.

I checked into a place called Sierra Tucson, in Arizona. I was actually excited about it, as I was eager to learn about alcoholism and the rehabilitation process, and about myself. It started off mundanely enough. The compound was peaceful and the grounds were well kept. Inside, the facility was clean and air-conditioned to a temperature that I really liked. When I checked in, they took everything I had that had alcohol in it—mouthwash, rubbing alcohol, anything. They led me to the "detox room," which was filled with incoming patients. In a bed to one side of me was a guy who appeared to be in his early twenties. He was deeply unconscious, and at first I thought he was dead. On the other side was a businessman who, I found out later, owned one of the largest air-conditioner companies in the world. His family had coordinated an intervention in which they tied him up, dressed him in a straitjacket, put him on his jet plane, and checked him into rehab.

Ten minutes after I was admitted, a doctor walked into the room, looked over at the young guy next to me, scribbled some notes on his chart, and moved on. He stopped at the millionaire businessman's bed and was like, "I'll get back to you." Finally, he walked over to me and asked me a series of questions about my vitals, each time looking down at his chart to record my answers. "How tall are you?" "How much do you weigh?"

He looked up at me and asked, "So when was the last time you had a drink?"

"A month ago," I replied straightforwardly.

He stared at me like I was nuts. I explained that I knew I was coming to rehab so, to prepare myself, I stopped drinking for the entire month of March. He grinned quickly and said, "You don't need to be in this room. Hold on a minute." He left the room for a few minutes. When he returned, he said, "You don't need to see me. Get your belongings, they'll show you to your room." They showed me where I would be staying. I met my roommate, a nice guy named Marco, who, I sadly found out, committed suicide years later.

The next morning, I went down to the psychologists' offices and the process started rolling. The psychologist began by rattling off a list of questions before explaining to me that the goal of Sierra Tucson was not just to get me off alcohol. The staff wanted me to understand the physical and biological reasons for substance abuse. They also aimed to delve into the psychological aspects of my alcoholism. They explained that the purpose wasn't just for me to stop drinking, but to learn *why* I was drinking in the first place.

She handed me a packet of things to read, which included four papers and some essays, and a stack of books. "You have to complete these before you leave," she said.

I had almost all of it done within the first two weeks of my stay.

It wasn't long before most of the other patients at the facility recognized me. They were shocked that I was there. The doctors and administrators offered to tell people to leave me alone, but that's the last thing I wanted. First off, being recognized has always come with the territory for me, so I was accustomed to people staring and asking questions. More important, I wasn't in any way trying to put on airs. I said, "No, don't tell anyone that, because this is part of who I am. I'm an alcoholic, too. I don't want to come in here like I'm someone special or above everyone else. They can come take pictures, they can ask me a million questions if they want to, I don't want to interrupt the process." I felt that, because I was DMC, I might be able to show the other patients that they had no reason to be ashamed of their situation or think that they were weak.

My doctors knew me, too, and because of that, they were able to ask questions that zeroed in on my experiences as part of Run-DMC. One of my therapists, after he learned who I was, asked, "Were there ever any instances in your career where Run or Russell or Jay or other group members did something that bothered you?"

I barely even thought about the question before I quickly responded, "Nope. Never."

He peered at me from above his eyeglasses and prodded me some more: "Come on, come on, you can be truthful."

"No," I insisted. "Everything was OK."

He sat there for a while, quiet, looking at me with his head tilted down. Then he lifted his head and looked me squarely in my eyes. "You're a goddamn liar!"

As surprised as I was by his response, I cracked up. It was the realest shit ever. I felt like I was back around the way in Hollis, Queens, he kept it so real. And since he was, I had to keep it real, too. So I came clean. I told him about all the times over the past twenty years when I had been bothered by all the things that had happened to me and around me. I told him how I had felt rejected, ignored, and misunderstood. When I finished, he said, "See, that's why you run to the bottle." He helped me see that I had been suppressing my emotions out of fear that, if I spoke my mind, I'd hurt someone else's feelings or would cause others to see me differently.

"D.," he went on, "you're so concerned about other

people that you're forgetting that the first person that you need to be concerned about is you. By you holding in all of your emotions, you'll go drink forty ounces of Olde English and other types of liquor, because you don't know how to deal with the feelings that you are going through." He sounded a lot like my wife right then.

As good as I thought alcohol made me feel, I learned that alcohol is actually a depressant. When I drank those 40s, they weren't helping remove the painful feelings, thoughts, and emotions I was experiencing. The alcohol only allowed me to force them further down into my psyche. "Things could have been totally different if you would have just spoken up," he explained. His words changed me. Ever since then, whether it hurts another person's feelings or not, I have to speak my truth. Now I speak my piece, no matter what it is.

I learned other valuable lessons in rehab, too. At one of my first classes, I was introduced to the twelve characteristics of an addictive personality. After the therapist wrote them on a board, he asked the group whether any of us saw anything on the list that pertained to us. I realized that I had, to varying degrees, all of those characteristics. Later, I also learned that I suffered from OCD—obsessive-compulsive disorder. All my life, I've had to have things in a certain type of order. All the labels on my food have to be facing outward. My clothes and shoes have to be lined up in a particular manner. I even stack all my coins into neat columns, quarters with quarters, nickels with nickels, dimes with dimes.

I used to think I was just a neat freak. But really, that kind of behavior is about control. I came to realize that I would drink whenever I didn't feel in control. I came to understand that nobody can control everything in life—and most certainly not other people.

I also learned to get rid of my excuses. As I say now, "Excuses don't explain and explanations don't excuse." I learned how to look in the mirror and face myself, my issues, my truths. I had spent too much of my life focusing on the wrong targets and then coming up with bullshit answers to excuse why things didn't work out. It's detrimental, not just to me but to others, when I don't speak the truth and face things as they really are. When I don't express what I am feeling, what I am thinking, what I am doing, then I do a disservice to myself and to others, because then we're all living a lie. And if that's the case, if I'm suppressing my emotions and feelings, how will the other person's feelings emerge? How will he or she find his or her own truth? Focusing on the wrong target leads far too many of us to turn to abusing substances, others, and even ourselves. We run from ourselves. In rehab, we're supposed to end up where we started, with nobody else but ourselves and, hopefully, with an entirely different view of who we are. I was able to see the person who was there all along, the person who was being suppressed.

Rehab was a version of the college experience. I learned. I engaged with others and shared whatever I had to offer. I took classes like Drama. I even performed an acoustic version of "Just Like Me" as part of a self-expression exercise. I had all the other patients coming to me privately trying to talk to me, and not because I was famous, but because of my outlook. They'd say I saw things differently. There I am in therapy, and I'm actually helping other people even as I'm being helped. It wasn't easy, but it was one of the most rewarding months of my life.

When I left, I didn't feel like I'd "fixed" someone who was broken. I wasn't broken. I just had had no idea who I was or why I did what I did. I left as myself, with the tools and the desire to now be the very best version of myself that I could be. I left ready to find out as much about myself as possible.

Now I was sober and armed with a healthy, new perspective. Therapy was my launching pad to the next stage of my life. Therapy made me less afraid of what the future would hold. Because I know I'm more than just a name on an album cover, that I have more value than just whatever profit I can help a record label earn, I can embrace the new phases that my life has seen. The last few years have represented both closure and a new beginning.

It's been an interesting journey, my passage from emotional turmoil to the peaceful and honest place I occupy now. It's been long and hard, fueled by fear and anger and, later, love. It's taken me to places I could've never imagined visiting, both out in the world and within my own soul. It's like I've come full circle, running away from myself, then returning better than when I started.

I'm probably more energetic than I was when I was younger, just because I was drunk all the time back then. Performing has never been an issue for me, whether sober or intoxicated, happy or depressed, but I'd be lying if I said it was easier to get on that stage drunk, overweight, and weighed down with all the emotional baggage I toted for the bulk of my career. I'm leaner now. My mind is clearer. My soul is unburdened. I have never in my life felt more potent as a performer.

Meanwhile, for the first time, I'm as healthy on the inside as on the outside. I'm done with chronic depression and thoughts of suicide. I'm no longer counting down the minutes before I can get offstage or out of a recording booth to go have a drink. I have worked through the pain I used to numb myself to avoid. I no longer feel like I have to endure people who are manipulative and unsupportive; I just cut them out of my life. Likewise, I don't worry anymore about losing friendships or love just because I made a choice that was good for me. I don't worry about who will get angry if I say no to something. I don't let people discount my feelings about matters either. I no longer wait for anybody to validate my opinions or affirm my good ideas. I'm secure enough now to know that doesn't matter.

This isn't to say I don't still struggle with problems. I do. I still find myself tensing up sometimes if I'm in the presence of people who I know don't have my best interests at heart. I have a very difficult time being around former friends who have let me down repeatedly over the years. I'm still inclined to retreat into my shell rather than hash out a conflict with someone—but now I brush off those inclinations and wade headlong into interpersonal difficulties. If we are going to have to work out a problem, then I'd rather we all be forced to deal with it, rather than just me. Back in the day, if there was a problem, I was prone to acting like it didn't matter and then drinking away whatever negative feelings I was masking.

I am a much better man now.

I thought about my journey recently when, around Christmas 2014, I found myself back onstage in New York, at the Barclays Center in Brooklyn, standing next to Run. It marked one of the few occasions we had performed together since we'd gone our separate ways in 2002. It was the first time since 1988 that Run-DMC had played New York.

I couldn't believe it had been that long, but it had. It was a milestone in its own right, marking for me not just where I'd come from, but also how far I had journeyed to get back to where I discovered my gift. It closed a circle on the one hand, but, on the other, it also represented the fact that I'd broken a cycle and found peace and prosperity in seeking my own direction. I wasn't the same DMC who'd ripped Madison Square Garden in 1986 and helped turn hip-hop into a commercial force. But on that Brooklyn stage that night, I was an artist who got a chance to study the impact of his handiwork. We could always do more, always be better. But sometimes it's satisfying just to know that the music that I discovered in the schoolyard of Saint Pascal's and the park jams of Hollis and the cafeteria tables at Rice High School is still going strong. Hip-hop has made a journey, too, is still traveling. I don't know exactly where it's going to end up, but I do know that it's got to keep moving to find out. Just like me.

My birth mother came to the show. It was the first time she'd ever seen me perform. On a New York stage as part of Run-DMC for the first time in almost twenty years, I was able to show her just what I had done with the opportunity she'd given me. She was right down front the whole time. When I gave her a shout-out, the crowd erupted in applause. I was sober. After decades of doubt and depression, I was whole. It feels good to be alive.

ACKNOWLEDGMENTS

Rock 'n' roll saved my soul, so I pray to the only god that I know!

Big hugs of love to my family, the Griffins and the McDanielses. There would be no Christmas in Hollis without y'all! No holidays or cookouts. Those were the most memorable events of my life!

Can't forget to acknowledge the real true pioneers of hip-hop, the people who touched and changed my life forever: Kool Herc and the Herculoids; Afrika Bambaataa and the Zulu Nation; Grandmaster Flash and the Furious Five; Grand Wizard Theodore and the Fantastic Five; DJs Breakout and Baron; the Funky Four Plus One More; the Treacherous Three; the Crash Crew; Dr. Rock and the

Force MCs; and my dudes Charlie Chase and Tony Tone and the Cold Crushin', Muthafuckin' Tough-Ass Four MCs!

Can't forget my solo faves DJ Hollywood, Lovebug Starski, Spoonie Gee, and Busy Bee!

And all the other pioneering MCs, DJs, break-dancers, and graffiti artists from the best era ever!

Love 'n' hugs to my Felix Organization family and Queen Mother Sheila Jaffe. You made it all possible!

Thank you, Erik Blam and Tracey Miller, for not abandoning ship when everyone else did.

To Trice, Charlie Chan, Bizkitt, Runny Ray, Smith, and Jesse Itzler for not being afraid to get back in the boat.

Thank you, Riggs and Ed, for adding another boat to the fleet! We're making the universe a better place.

To Shawnee and Johnny Warfield and my BrandFire buddies for making dreams come true. It's on!

Most important, I would like to acknowledge all or-phans, foster kids, adoptees, and anyone going through any battles with alcohol, drugs, and any other substances.

To all people going through anything emotional, physical, or spiritual, remember this:

You are not alone!

ABOUT THE AUTHOR

Darryl "DMC" McDaniels is a musical icon and one of the founders—along with Joseph "Rev. Run" Simmons and the late, great Jason "Jam Master Jay" Mizell—of the ground-breaking rap group Run-DMC. With a fan base that rivals some of the biggest acts in rock and roll, Run-DMC has sold more than thirty million singles and albums world-wide and has helped transform rap and hip-hop into one of the most popular musical genres of all time. In 2009, the group was inducted into the Rock and Roll Hall of Fame. In 2014, McDaniels launched the comic book company Darryl Makes Comics and published the graphic novel *DMC*. His work with the Felix Organization, a nonprofit he cofounded, led him to speak at the White House and appear before Congress and various state legislatures on behalf of adoptees and foster children. When he's not on tour speaking or performing, he lives in New York City.